Lecture Notes in Mechanical Engineering

Lecture Notes in Mechanical Engineering (LNME) publishes the latest developments in Mechanical Engineering—quickly, informally and with high quality. Original research or contributions reported in proceedings and post-proceedings represents the core of LNME. Volumes published in LNME embrace all aspects, subfields and new challenges of mechanical engineering.

To submit a proposal or request further information, please contact the Springer Editor of your location:

Europe, USA, Africa: Leontina Di Cecco at Leontina.dicecco@springer.com
China: Ella Zhang at ella.zhang@cn.springernature.com
India, Rest of Asia, Australia, New Zealand: Swati Meherishi at swati.meherishi@springer.com

Topics in the series include:

- Engineering Design
- Machinery and Machine Elements
- Mechanical Structures and Stress Analysis
- Automotive Engineering
- Engine Technology
- Aerospace Technology and Astronautics
- Nanotechnology and Microengineering
- Control, Robotics, Mechatronics
- MEMS
- Theoretical and Applied Mechanics
- Dynamical Systems, Control
- Fluid Mechanics
- Engineering Thermodynamics, Heat and Mass Transfer
- Manufacturing Engineering and Smart Manufacturing
- Precision Engineering, Instrumentation, Measurement
- Materials Engineering
- Tribology and Surface Technology

Indexed by SCOPUS, EI Compendex, and INSPEC.

All books published in the series are evaluated by Web of Science for the Conference Proceedings Citation Index (CPCI).

To submit a proposal for a monograph, please check our Springer Tracts in Mechanical Engineering at https://link.springer.com/bookseries/11693.

Filip Górski · Răzvan Păcurar · Nikola Vitković ·
Michał Rychlik · Michał Jakubowicz
Editors

Advances in Manufacturing V

Volume 5 - Biomedical Engineering: Factory of the Future

Springer

Editors
Filip Górski
Faculty of Mechanical Engineering
Poznań University of Technology
Poznań, Poland

Nikola Vitković
Faculty of Mechanical Engineering
University of Niš
Niš, Serbia

Michał Jakubowicz
Faculty of Mechanical Engineering
Poznań University of Technology
Poznań, Poland

Răzvan Păcurar
Manufacturing Engineering Department
Technical University of Cluj-Napoca
Cluj-Napoca, Romania

Michał Rychlik
Faculty of Mechanical Engineering
Poznań University of Technology
Poznań, Poland

ISSN 2195-4356 ISSN 2195-4364 (electronic)
Lecture Notes in Mechanical Engineering
ISBN 978-3-032-23088-1 ISBN 978-3-032-23089-8 (eBook)
https://doi.org/10.1007/978-3-032-23089-8

This Springer imprint is published by the registered company Springer Nature Switzerland AG
The registered company address is: Gewerbestrasse 11, 6330 Cham, Switzerland

Preface

This volume of Lecture Notes in Mechanical Engineering gathers accepted papers presented at the 9th International Scientific-Technical Conference MANUFACTURING 2026, held in Poznan, Poland on May 19–21, 2026. The conference was hosted by the Faculty of Mechanical Engineering, Poznan University of Technology, Poland.

The primary objective of the MANUFACTURING 2026 was to showcase cutting-edge advancements across the broad spectrum of mechanical engineering, providing a dynamic forum for the exchange of innovative ideas and expert opinions. Focused on the theme of the Factory of the Future, the conference serves as a vital platform for dialogue on industrial evolution and science-industry synergy. Its global reach continues to expand, as evidenced by the consistently increasing participation from international research centers. Furthermore, the event fosters the integration of academia with the economic sector, encouraging collaboration with industry leaders and management professionals interested in implementing research results into business practice. The scope encompassed the following areas:

- Mechanical Engineering
- Production Engineering
- Quality Engineering
- Measurement and Control Systems
- Biomedical Engineering

The global significance of the conference is reflected in the diversity of the submissions. The Organizing Committee received 219 contributions from 37 countries. To ensure the highest academic standards, all papers underwent a rigorous double-blind peer review process. Each manuscript was evaluated by at least three independent international experts, with a strict limit of five assignments per reviewer to guarantee depth and quality of feedback. Following this comprehensive appraisal, 120 papers were accepted for publication (an acceptance rate of 55%), representing the work of 347 authors from 25 countries. A total of 109 articles were published in the proceedings Advances in Manufacturing IV, while 11 selected papers appeared in the journal Management and Production Engineering Review, issued under the auspices of the Committee on Production Engineering of the Polish Academy of Sciences and the Polish Society for Production Management.

The review process focused on originality of paper, significance of presented results, comprehensibility and quality of the presentation, relevance for this conference and overall impression. Furthermore, reviewers meticulously assessed the timeliness of the research, the adequacy of the literature review, methodological rigor, and the clarity of conclusions, as well as the quality of English. Feedback provided to authors included specific recommendations for improving methodology, data presentation, and editorial quality. Acceptance required at least two positive reviews and a full resolution of all reviewers' concerns. This international effort involved experts from 30 countries across Europe, North America, South Asia, and North Africa. Additionally, all manuscripts were checked using anti-plagiarism software, which allowed the similarity index to be less than 15%.

The book **Advances in Manufacturing V** is organized into five volumes that correspond to the main conference disciplines mentioned above.

The **Advances in Manufacturing V – Volume 5 – Biomedical Engineering: Factory of the Future** volume focuses on the paradigm shift toward the Factory of the Future regarding design and production of medical devices and services. The volume presents a collection of scientific papers focused on the transformation of biomedical engineering in the era of intelligent, data-driven, and digitally integrated healthcare manufacturing. The contributions address the convergence of advanced design, modeling, and fabrication technologies that are redefining how medical devices and products are conceived, customized, and produced. The content is structured into four thematic parts, reflecting the multidisciplinary nature of modern biomedical engineering.

Section I: Digital Design, Modeling, and Intelligent Systems in Biomedical Engineering. This section establishes the digital intelligence layer - AI-assisted interaction, parametric anatomy-driven modeling, and VR-based digital twins, which underpins future biomedical manufacturing and education.

Section II: Intelligent and Automated Manufacturing Systems for Medical Applications. These contributions address process accuracy, robotic integration, and virtual validation, directly reflecting the Factory of the Future concept applied to medical production environments.

Section III: Patient-Specific Implants, Prostheses, and Orthotic Devices. This section showcases end-use medical devices, emphasizing customization, functional validation, and user-centered design, key outcomes of digital biomedical manufacturing.

Section IV: Advanced Materials, Characterization, and Performance Validation in Medical Additive Manufacturing. This section addresses the materials and validation layer of the Factory of the Future, linking bioactivity, mechanical reliability, and next-generation AM materials to clinical performance.

Comprising 14 chapters prepared by 56 authors from 8 countries, this volume provides valuable insights and practical perspectives for professionals, academics, and innovators shaping the future of biomedical engineering and medical product manufacturing, fostering a vital synergy between science, healthcare and industry.

We wish to express our sincere gratitude to the members of the Scientific and Program Committees for their dedication and expertise during the review process. We also extend our thanks to the authors, sponsors, and all contributors whose commitment was instrumental in making MANUFACTURING 2026 a resounding success.

May 2026

Filip Górski
Răzvan Păcurar
Nikola Vitković
Michał Rychlik
Michał Jakubowicz

Organization

Steering Committee

General Chair

Adam Hamrol	Poznan University of Technology, Poland

Chairs

Bartosz Gapiński	Poznan University of Technology, Poland
Magdalena Hryb	Poznan University of Technology, Poland
Justyna Trojanowska	Poznan University of Technology, Poland

Conference Founders

Zenobia Weiss (Deceased)	Poznan University of Technology, Poland
Adam Hamrol	Poznan University of Technology, Poland

Scientific Committee

Katarzyna Antosz	Rzeszow University of Technology, Poland
Christopher Brown	Worcester Polytechnic Institute, USA
Anna Burduk	Wrocław University of Science and Technology, Poland
Suthep Butdee	Rajamangala University of Technology Krungthep, Thailand
Marcin Butlewski	Poznan University of Technology, Poland
Olaf Ciszak	Poznan University of Technology, Poland
Reggie Davidrajuh	University of Stavanger, Norway
Ewa Dostatni	Poznan University of Technology, Poland
Jan Duda	Cracow University of Technology, Poland
Mosè Gallo	University of Naples Federico II, Italy
Bartosz Gapiński	Poznan University of Technology, Poland
Józef Gawlik	Cracow University of Technology, Poland
Adam Gąska	Cracow University of Technology, Poland

Arkadiusz Gola	Lublin University of Technology, Poland
Filip Górski	Poznan University of Technology, Poland
Marta Grabowska	Poznan University of Technology, Poland
Adam Hamrol	Poznan University of Technology, Poland
Magdalena Hryb	Poznan University of Technology, Poland
Jozef Husár	Technical University of Košice, Slovakia
Aminul Islam	Technical University of Denmark, Denmark
Vitalii Ivanov	Sumy State University, Ukraine
Michał Jakubowicz	Poznan University of Technology, Poland
Andrzej Jardzioch	West Pomeranian University of Technology in Szczecin, Poland
Sabahudin Jasarevic	University of Zenica, Bosnia & Herzegovina
Małgorzata Jasiulewicz-Kaczmarek	Poznan University of Technology, Poland
Anna Karwasz	Poznan University of Technology, Poland
Sławomir Kłos	Poznan University of Technology, Poland
Lucia Knapčíková	Technical University of Košice, Slovakia
Agnieszka Kujawińska	Poznan University of Technology, Poland
Vijaya Kumar Manupati	National Institute of Industrial Engineering, India
Stanisław Legutko	Poznan University of Technology, Poland
Sławomir Luściński	Kielce University of Technology, Poland
José Machado	University of Minho, Portugal
Damjan Maletic	University of Maribor, Slovenia
Dariusz Mikołajewski	Kazimierz Wielki University, Poland
Piotr Moncarz	Stanford University, USA
Magdalena Niemczewska-Wójcik	Cracow University of Technology, Poland
Przemysław Niewiadomski	University of Zielona Góra, Poland
Razvan Ioan Pacurar	Technical University of Cluj-Napoca, Romania
Piotr Paczos	Poznan University of Technology, Poland
Mirosław Pajor	Maritime University of Szczecin, Poland
Justyna Patalas-Maliszewska	University of Zielona Góra, Poland
Ivan Pavlenko	Sumy State University, Ukraine
Erwin Rauch	Free University of Bozen-Bolzano, Italy
Paulina Rewers	Poznan University of Technology, Poland
Izabela Rojek	Kazimierz Wielki University, Poland
Michał Rychlik	Poznan University of Technology, Poland
Krzysztof Santarek	Warsaw University of Technology, Poland
Sebastian Skoczypiec	Cracow University of Technology, Poland
Bożena Skołud	Silesian University of Technology, Poland
Jerzy Andrzej Sładek	Cracow University of Technology, Poland
Beata Starzyńska	Poznan University of Technology, Poland

Liangyan Tao	Nanjing University of Aeronautics and Astronautics, China
Anna Timofiejczuk	Silesian University of Technology, Poland
Justyna Trojanowska	Poznan University of Technology, Poland
Wiesław Urban	Bialystok University of Technology, Poland
Leonilde Varela	University of Minho, Portugal
Nikola Vitković	University of Niš, Serbia
Michał Wieczorowski	Poznan University of Technology, Poland
Ewa Więcek-Janka	Poznan University of Technology, Poland
Szymon Wojciechowski	Poznan University of Technology, Poland
Ralf Woll	BTU Cottbus-Senftenberg, Germany
Naiming Xie	Nanjing University of Aeronautics and Astronautics, China
Jiehan Zhou	Shandong University of Science and Technology, China

Program Committee

Adam Gąska	Cracow University of Technology, Poland
Adam Hamrol	Poznan University of Technology, Poland
Agnieszka Kaczmarek-Pawelska	University of Zielona Góra, Poland
Agnieszka Stachowiak	Poznan University of Technology, Poland
Alejandro Pereira	University of Vigo, Portugal
Aleksandar Miltenovic	University of Nis, Serbia
Alice Chlupová	Czech Academy of Sciences, Czech Republic
Alzbeta Sapietova	University of Žilina, Slovakia
Ancuta Pacurar	Technical University of Cluj-Napoca, Romania
André Guimarães	University of Beira Interior, Portugal
Andrzej Jardzioch	West Pomeranian University of Technology in Szczecin, Poland
Angelika Hofer	Free University of Bozen-Bolzano, Italy
Anna Borucka	Military University of Technology Warsaw, Poland
Anna Burduk	Wroclaw University of Science and Technology, Poland
Anna Karwasz	Poznan University of Technology, Poland
Anna M. Deptuła	Opole University of Technology, Poland
Anna Saniuk	University of Zielona Góra, Poland
Arkadiusz Gola	Lublin University of Technology, Poland
Bartosz Gapinski	Poznan University of Technology, Poland
Bogdan Dybała	Wroclaw University of Science and Technology, Poland

Christopher Brown	Worcester Polytechnic Institute, USA
Cristina Stefana Miron-Borzan	Technical University of Cluj-Napoca, Romania
Dagmara Łapczyńska	Wroclaw University of Science and Technology, Poland
Damian Grajewski	Poznan University of Technology, Poland
Damian Krenczyk	Silesian University of Technology, Poland
Dan-Sorin Comsa	Technical University of Cluj-Napoca, Romania
Daniel Medyński	Witelon Collegium State University, Poland
Dariusz Mikołajewski	Kazimierz Wielki University, Poland
Djahida Belayadi	National School of Cybersecurity, Algeria
Dražan Kozak	University of Slavonski Brod, Croatia
Edward Kozłowski	Lublin University of Technology, Poland
Emilia Campean	Technical University of Cluj-Napoca, Romania
Emilia Sabau	Technical University of Cluj-Napoca, Romania
Eryk Szwarc	Koszalin University of Technology, Poland
Ewa Dostatni	Poznan University of Technology, Poland
Ewa Więcek-Janka	Poznan University of Technology, Poland
Gabriel Stolárik	Technical University of Košice, Slovakia
Grzegorz Pająk	University of Zielona Góra, Poland
Hanna Łosyk	University of Zielona Góra, Poland
Hubert Wojciechowski	Poznan University of Technology, Poland
Izabela Kudelska	Poznan University of Technology, Poland
Izabela Rojek	Kazimierz Wielki University, Poland
Jacek Diakun	Poznan University of Technology, Poland
Jakub Kaščák	Technical University of Košice, Slovakia
Jakub Kopowski	Kazimierz Wielki University, Poland
Jerzy Jozwik	Lublin University of Technology, Poland
Joanna Cyganiuk	University of Zielona Góra, Poland
Joanna Helman	Wroclaw University of Science and Technology, Poland
Joanna Wilczarska	Bydgoszcz University of Science and Technology, Poland
Jozef Husár	Technical University of Košice, Slovakia
Jozef Török	Technical University of Košice, Slovakia
Józef Kuczmaszewski	Lublin University of Technology, Poland
Justyna Patalas-Maliszewska	University of Zielona Góra, Poland
Kamil Krot	Wroclaw University of Science and Technology, Poland
Kamil Leksycki	University of Zielona Góra, Poland
Kamil Musiał	Wroclaw University of Science and Technology, Poland
Karol Dąbrowski	University of Zielona Góra, Poland

Katarzyna Antosz	Rzeszow University of Technology, Poland
Katarzyna Cheba	West Pomeranian University of Technology in Szczecin, Poland
Katarzyna Kazimierska-Drobny	Kazimierz Wielki University, Poland
Katarzyna Skrzypek	University of Zielona Góra, Poland
Khrystyna Berladir	Sumy State University, Ukraine
Konrad Kobiela	Cracow University of Technology, Poland
Krzysztof Kalinowski	Silesian University of Technology, Poland
Krzysztof Nowacki	Silesian University of Technology, Poland
Krzysztof Żywicki	Poznan University of Technology, Poland
Leonilde Varela	University of Minho, Portugal
Lucia Knapčíková	Technical University of Košice, Slovakia
Łukasz Rymaniak	Poznan University of Technology, Poland
Magdalena Hryb	Poznan University of Technology, Poland
Magdalena Rybaczewska-Błażejowska	Kielce University of Technology, Poland
Magdalena Żukowska	Poznan University of Technology, Poland
Małgorzata Śliwa	University of Zielona Góra, Poland
Marcin Suszynski	Poznan University of Technology, Poland
Marek Kočiško	Technical University of Košice, Slovakia
Marek Macko	Kazimierz Wielki University, Poland
Maria Rosienkiewicz	Wroclaw University of Science and Technology, Poland
Marian Bartoszuk	Opole University of Technology, Poland
Marius Sorin Pustan	Technical University of Cluj-Napoca, Romania
Marks Gorohovs	Riga Technical University, Latvia
Marta Grabowska	Poznan University of Technology, Poland
Marta Harničárová	Slovak University of Agriculture in Nitra, Slovakia
Michał Jakubowicz	Poznan University of Technology, Poland
Michał Rogalewicz	Poznan University of Technology, Poland
Mihai Dragomir	Technical University of Cluj-Napoca, Romania
Milan Edl	Univcrsity of Wcst Bohcmia, Czcch Rcpublic
Mircea Fulea	Technical University of Cluj-Napoca, Romania
Mukund Harugade	Padmabhooshan Vasantraodada Patil Institute of Technology, India
Natalya Shramenko	Lviv Polytechnic National University, Ukraine
Nataša Náprstková	University of Jan Evangelista in Ústí nad Labem, Czech Republic
Nguyen Hong Vi	Vietnamese German University, Vietnam
Nikola Vitković	University of Nis, Serbia
Olaf Ciszak	Poznan University of Technology, Poland

Olha Kalman	Technical University of Košice, Slovakia
Paulina Rewers	Poznan University of Technology, Poland
Paweł Buń	Poznan University of Technology, Poland
Paweł Szczygieł	Kielce University of Technology, Poland
Paweł Zmarzły	Kielce University of Technology, Poland
Pedro Torres	Polytechnic Institute of Castelo Branco, Portugal
Piotr Gąska	AGH University of Krakow, Poland
Piotr Kotlarz	Kazimierz Wielki University, Poland
Piotr Trojanowski	West Pomeranian University of Technology in Szczecin, Poland
Piotr Ziembicki	University of Zielona Góra, Poland
Przemysław Zawadzki	Poznan University of Technology, Poland
Radosław Wichniarek	Poznan University of Technology, Poland
Răzvan Păcurar	Technical University of Cluj-Napoca, Romania
Roman Kielec	University of Zielona Góra, Poland
Sandra Grabowska	Silesian University of Technology, Poland
Sebastian Saniuk	University of Zielona Góra, Poland
Sebastian Skoczypiec	Cracow University of Technology, Poland
Sergej Hloch	Technical University of Košice, Slovakia
Sławomir Kłos	University of Zielona Góra, Poland
Stanislaw Legutko	Poznan University of Technology, Poland
Stella Hrehova	Technical University of Košice, Slovakia
Sven Maricic	Juraj Dobrila University of Pula, Croatia
Sylvia Kusmierczak	University of Jan Evangelista in Ústí nad Labem, Czech Republic
Szymon Wojciechowski	Poznan University of Technology, Poland
Thanh Tran	RMIT University, Vietnam
Tomasz Bednarek	Kazimierz Wielki University, Poland
Vijaya Kumar Manupati	NITIE Mumbai, India
Vitalii Ivanov	Sumy State University, Ukraine
Wiesław Kuczko	Poznan University of Technology, Poland
Wiktor Szot	Kielce University of Technology, Poland
Wojciech Babirecki	University of Zielona Góra, Poland
Wojciech Macek	Gdańsk University of Technology, Poland
Yuliia Denysenko	Sumy State University, Ukraine
Zbigniew Wiśniewski	Lodz University of Technology, Poland
Zuzana Mitaľová	Technical University of Košice, Slovakia

Special Sessions and Special Session Organizing Committee

Efficiency-Driven Manufacturing: Tools and Trends in the Era of Industry 4.0

Justyna Trojanowska	Poznan University of Technology, Poland
Leonilde Varela	University of Minho, Portugal
Vijaya Kumar Manupati	NITIE Mumbai, India
Thanh Tran	RMIT University, Vietnam
Jozef Husár	Technical University of Košice, Slovakia

Intersecting Quality Management and Mechanical Design for Manufacturing Sustainability

Florin Popişter	Technical University of Cluj-Napoca, Romania
Diana Cristina Dragomir	Technical University of Cluj-Napoca, Romania
Corina Julieta Birleanu	Technical University of Cluj-Napoca, Romania
Mircea Claudiu Fulea	Technical University of Cluj-Napoca, Romania

Human Factors in Manufacturing

Marcin Butlewski	Poznan University of Technology, Poland
Beata Mrugalska	Poznan University of Technology, Poland
Wiktoria Czernecka	Poznan University of Technology, Poland
Fryderyk Wachowiak	Poznan University of Technology, Poland
Krzysztof Hankiewicz	Poznan University of Technology, Poland

Circularity in Advanced Production Systems: Materials, Methods, and Digital Transformation

Marek Kočisko	Technical University of Košice, Slovakia
Lucia Knapčikova	Technical University of Košice, Slovakia
Jakub Kaščak	Technical University of Košice, Slovakia
Jozef Török	Technical University of Košice, Slovakia

Smart Manufacturing and Sustainability: Interdisciplinary Approaches in the Era of Industry 4.0/5.0

From Additive Manufacturing to Healthcare Innovation through Digital Transformation in Biomedical Engineering

Intelligent Adaptive Systems in Integrated Production Management Processes

Intelligent Solutions for Industry of the Future

Grey Systems Modeling for Engineering Solutions and Business Optimization

Magdalena Hryb	Poznan University of Technology, Poland
Agnieszka Kujawińska	Poznan University of Technology, Poland
Naiming Xie	Nanjing University of Aeronautics and Astronautics, China
Liangyan Tao	Nanjing University of Aeronautics and Astronautics, China
Rafał Mierzwiak	Poznan University of Technology, Poland

Intelligent Methods Supporting Manufacturing Systems Efficiency

Anna Burduk	Wroclaw University of Science and Technology, Poland
Damian Krenczyk	Silesian University of Technology, Poland
Dagmara Łapczyńska	Wroclaw University of Science and Technology, Poland
Kamil Krot	Wroclaw University of Science and Technology, Poland

Contents

Patient-Specific Implants, Prostheses, and Orthotic Devices

Advanced Materials, Characterization, and Performance Validation in Medical Additive Manufacturing

Digital Design, Modeling, and Intelligent Systems in Biomedical Engineering

VR Simulation and Education for Additive Manufacturing in Medicine: A Process-Oriented Engineering Approach

Nikola Vitković[1(✉)], Aleksandar Trajkovic[1], Rajko Turudija[1], Jovan Arandjelovic[1], Monica Maria Elena Rauca[2], and Diana Elena Horincar[2]

[1] Faculty of Mechanical Engineering, University of Nis, Niš, Serbia
nikola.vitkovic@masfak.ni.ac.rs
[2] Technical University of Cluj-Napoca, Cluj-Napoca, Romania

Abstract. Virtual Reality (VR) and Additive Manufacturing (AM) are transforming modern engineering education, especially in biomedical engineering fields where precision, customization, and collaboration across disciplines are essential. This paper introduces a process-focused framework that combines A-Frame, an open-source WebXR platform for immersive, browser-based simulations, with CALLME, an AI-supported educational tool. The integrated system enables students to explore and analyze every phase of the AM process, modeling, slicing, fabrication, and inspection, within a VR laboratory directly connected to CALLME's adaptive analytics. The aim is to enhance the understanding of AM concepts through interactive digital twins, real-time feedback on parameters, and measurable learning outcomes. This approach promotes open, scalable, and data-driven education aligned with the human-centric principles of Industry 5.0. The achieved outcomes of the proposed framework include: (i) a structured, process-oriented representation of the complete additive manufacturing workflow in an immersive VR environment; (ii) real-time coupling of learner interactions with learning analytics, enabling objective observation of parameter exploration and decision-making strategies; and (iii) improved conceptual understanding of cause–effect relationships in AM processes through immediate visual feedback and adaptive learning paths.

Keywords: Virtual Reality · Additive Manufacturing · A-Frame · CALLME · AI

1 Introduction

Additive Manufacturing (AM) is one of the most transformative technologies in modern medicine, allowing for the creation of customized anatomical models, implants, and patient-specific devices. However, engineering education has not yet fully adapted to this shift. Traditional engineering education often separates CAD modeling, slicing, and production into isolated learning activities [1]. This fragmentation limits students' understanding of process dependencies across the additive manufacturing workflow [2]. VR provides a compelling solution. By simulating complete AM workflows,

F. Górski et al. (Eds.): MANUFACTURING 2026, LNME, pp. 3–11, 2026.
https://doi.org/10.1007/978-3-032-23089-8_1

students can experiment with parameters, observe real-time results, and understand process dependencies in a resource-efficient and environmentally sustainable manner, eliminating the need for physical trials. Modern WebXR frameworks, especially A-Frame, enable browser-based VR scenes accessible from any device, promoting inclusivity and scalability. This paper introduces an educational framework combining A-Frame and CALLME – "Collaborative e-platform for innovation and educational enhancement in medical engineering", where A-Frame offers immersive, process-focused simulations, and CALLME supplies analytics, adaptive feedback, and modular course structure. The integration is lightweight, reproducible, and suitable for blended and remote learning scenarios.

2 State of the Art

2.1 Additive Manufacturing Education

The evolution of AM education has not fully matched technological advances in the field. Early additive manufacturing curricula primarily focused on machine operation and rapid prototyping [3]. More recent educational approaches emphasize Design for Additive Manufacturing (DfAM), addressing design freedom, material behavior, and process limitations [1]. Sources in [2, 3] describe how the shift from rapid prototyping to functional production requires a multidisciplinary educational model linking digital design, process simulation, and sustainability.

A key development has been the introduction of virtual and hybrid laboratories. As reported in [4], significant gains occur when students practice parameter tuning and build-failure analysis virtually before working in real labs. Recent analyses note that AM education should balance hands-on skill development with a deep understanding of the digital workflow.

Modern AM curricula increasingly incorporate simulation-driven design, generative modeling, and process monitoring. Digital twins help students visualize cause-and-effect relationships between variables such as layer thickness, extrusion temperature, and print speed. These virtual tools, combined with intelligent learning environments, offer personalized learning paths and analytics on student interactions.

In biomedical applications, AM training intersects with anatomical modeling and patient-specific design. Here, spatial perception and process understanding are crucial: students must turn 3D medical images (CT/MRI) into printable anatomical models. These tasks require integrated training environments capable of visualizing geometry and biomechanical constraints [5]. Browser-based VR platforms provide ideal scalability for such instruction [6], and these efforts align with human-centric industry frameworks [7].

2.2 Virtual Reality in Engineering and Medical Training

VR has established itself as a catalyst for experiential learning. Virtual laboratories have been shown to support conceptual understanding in medical and engineering education [8]. Immersive virtual reality has been shown to significantly support conceptual understanding and knowledge retention by enabling active exploration and embodied cognition, compared to traditional screen-based instruction [9]. Browser-based VR environments further reduce technical barriers and cognitive overhead by simplifying access and interaction [6]. These effects are particularly relevant in medical education, where spatial reasoning plays a critical role [7]. Work in surgical and procedural training demonstrates improvements in skill transfer, procedural accuracy, and situational awareness that translates to machine operation and process optimization [10]. In biomedical engineering, immersive 3D visualization supports anatomical exploration, prosthetic fitting, and scaffold design, giving learners and practitioners intuitive control over spatial and process variables [5, 8, 9]. Systematic reviews of immersive VR applications in higher education indicate consistent benefits in learner engagement, motivation, and spatial understanding, particularly in technical and engineering disciplines [11].

Historically, high-quality VR environments require complex tool chains and dedicated hardware. The emergence of WebXR, and especially A-Frame, overcomes these challenges: declarative scene composition, easy distribution via the browser, and wide device compatibility [6]. This democratization of access supports remote learners, interdisciplinary teams, and institutions with limited resources. Moreover, combining VR with AI-guided learning yields adaptivity: interaction logs and simulation events can feed analytics to assess behavior, parameter exploration, and decision-making strategies, enabling timely remediation or advancement [12].

Modern education increasingly depends on learning analytics, adaptive systems, and personalization. CALLME connects pedagogy, analytics, and interactivity by organizing content into Knowledge Atoms (KAs), self-contained learning units with media, assessments, and external interactive modules, including VR. Each KA specifies competencies, outcomes, and analytics hooks. The AI components track time on tasks, interaction patterns, and parameter sequences to evaluate how successful the learning process is and adapt progression. Unlike traditional Learning Management Systems (LMSs), CALLME ingests real-time simulation data, providing behavioral analytics beyond quizzes. The platform exposes modular Application Programming Interfaces (APIs) for VR content, allowing easy embedding of A-Frame scenes within lessons [6, 12]. This integration aligns with human-centered principles of Industry 5.0 [7].

3 Methodology

3.1 Framework Architecture

The proposed framework (Fig. 1) links engineering simulation and educational analytics to establish a learning-by-doing environment in AM.

It consists of three complementary layers that function as a continuous feedback loop involving visualization, interaction, and evaluation:

- Engineering Process Layer: model preparation, slicing, production, and inspection, driven by variables such as layer height, nozzle temperature, extrusion speed, and infill density;
- VR Simulation Layer: an A-Frame WebXR environment visualizing printer kinematics, toolpath logic, and material deposition for perceiving spatial relationships and how digital parameters influence outcomes;

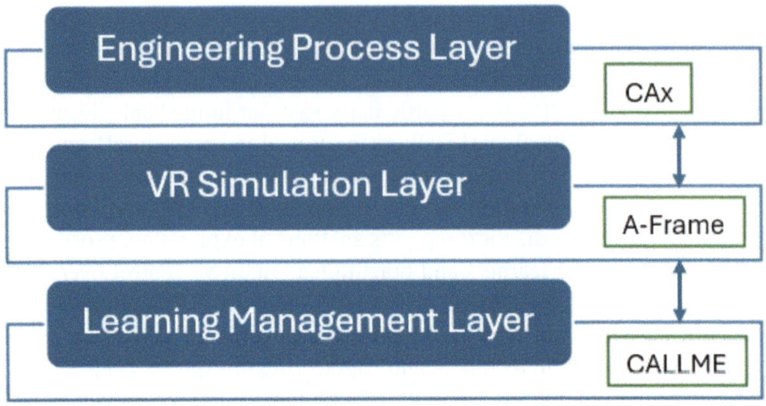

Fig. 1. Conceptual architecture linking A-Frame simulation with CALLME analytics.

- Learning Management Layer: CALLME organizes content into KAs, manages sessions and interactions, and uses adaptive analytics to create personalized learning pathways.

Together, these layers create a closed loop between action, reflection, and adaptation: what the student manipulates in VR is captured by the analytics engine, which refines future learning tasks.

The workflow links student interactions in VR with backend analytics in real time. Students select a 3D model and set process parameters (layer height, nozzle temperature, print speed, infill). CALLME packages parameters as structured JSON and sends them to the A-Frame scene via a RESTful API. The WebXR environment runs entirely in the browser, interpreting parameters to control motion and visual feedback. During simulation, events (start, pause, reset, parameter changes, layer complete, error detected) are timestamped and transmitted back to CALLME via HTTPS or WebSocket. CALLME aggregates these into learning vectors (interaction frequency, time on task, error recovery). An AI analytics engine identifies patterns, assesses knowledge retention, and updates adaptive progression. Learning analytics enable the analysis of learner behavior and interaction patterns in immersive environments [13]. Recent studies emphasize the role of immersive technologies in assessing procedural knowledge and skill development [14]. Such approaches have been increasingly applied in medical and technical education contexts [15].

3.2 A-Frame Implementation

The A-Frame implementation is made through visual and interactive cores. Built with HTML and JavaScript, it offers experiential richness with a lightweight stack. Following the Entity-Component-System paradigm, scene elements (printer frame, bed, gantry, nozzle and UI panel) are entities whose behaviors (motion, transformation, color response and interaction) are modular components, allowing extensions without altering the core, Figs. 2 and 3. Taking this into account, the design goal was pedagogical transparency. To achieve this, movements are scaled and smoothed for clarity rather than strict physical accuracy. Additionally, parameter-effect relationships are visual and immediate: speed modulates gantry motion, higher temperature changes nozzle color, and infill density appears via bead spacing.

Furthermore, the nozzle is modeled as a child of the gantry with offset compensation, so its tip consistently follows the bed plane through the build. Concerning parameter modeling and their integration with the UI: speed, temperature, and infill appear on a floating side panel as clickable controls with keyboard shortcuts (S = Start, P = Pause, R = Reset), making the printer model accessible.

When talking about visual semantics and performance, optimized primitives (a-box, a-cylinder and a-cone) sustain performance on low-end devices. Extruded material is represented through cylinders placed on the bed to depict layer formation. Concerning analytics, each user action dispatches an event captured for analytics without degrading performance. Importantly, the modular design allows for future extensions (dual nozzles, resin processes, importing toolpaths, etc.).

The main pedagogical focus is emphasized in conceptual understanding. Students test hypotheses and immediately observe results, with declarative scene edits enabling alignment to course objectives. The VR simulations are implemented using WebXR and are compatible with both PC-based VR setups (e.g., desktop or laptop with a standard browser) and standalone head-mounted displays such as Meta Quest devices, enabling flexible deployment across different educational environments.

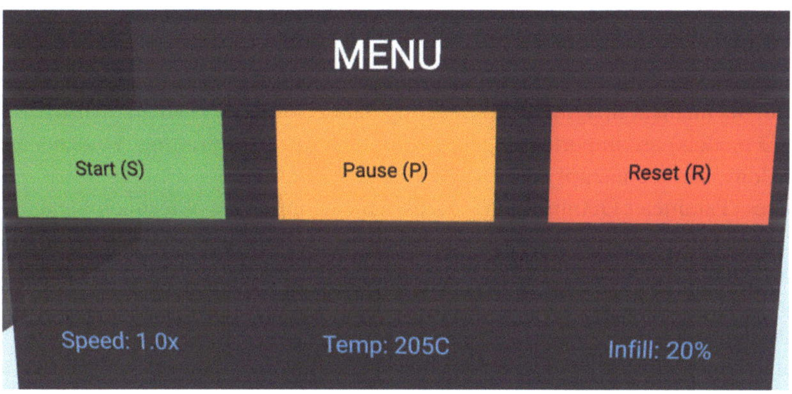

Fig. 2. The Educational scene of MENU in A-Frame

3.3 Communication and Integration with CALLME

Data exchange between VR and the backend uses standard HTTPS REST and WebSocket communication. The embedded A-Frame simulation transmits event logs in JSON and receives parameter configurations or task updates. Data is processed by AI-driven analytics and visualized on the portal. Integration relies on open protocols and lightweight components, enabling replication across institutions.

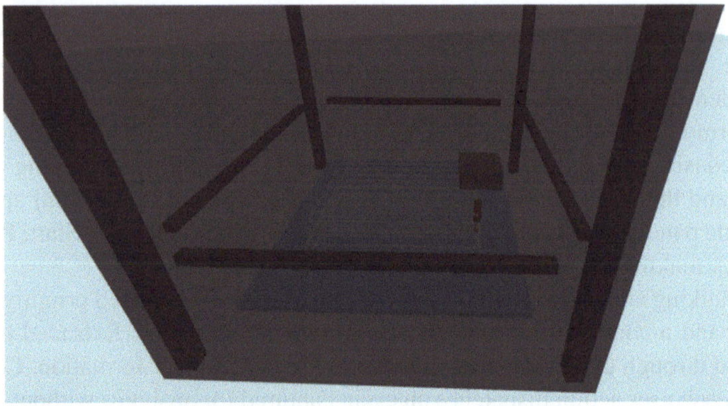

Fig. 3. The Educational scene in A-Frame

Each course within the CALLME platform (https://callmeed.net) is constructed as a structured sequence of KAs: compact, goal-driven learning units that interconnect theoretical, procedural, and experiential dimensions of education. This atomized design reflects a shift from monolithic course modules toward modular, data-rich learning ecosystems. Each KA integrates instructional content, interactive exercise, formative assessment, and analytics that together create a continuous learning-feedback loop.

In the context of AM education, CALLME organizes courses into a progression of thematically linked KAs that mirror real process stages:

- Model Preparation – introduces learners to geometric and anatomical modeling. Here, 3D medical imaging or engineering datasets (e.g., CT/MRI reconstructions or CAD models) are imported, segmented, and adapted for printing. Students analyze topology, surface integrity, and manufacturability criteria.
- Process Parameter Optimization – focuses on the influence of technological parameters such as layer height, nozzle temperature, print speed, and infill density. Within the embedded A-Frame simulation, users can manipulate these parameters and observe immediate visual feedback on toolpath generation, deposition quality, and build stability.
- Defect Analysis – trains learners to identify, categorize, and reduce printing errors such as warping, layer separation, and void formation. Simulation-driven diagnostic scenarios encourage analytical thinking and problem-solving.

Each KA can embed an A-Frame-based VR exercise that functions as an interactive laboratory within the CALLME environment. The simulation allows students to perform virtual experiments, adjusting process parameters, observing material behavior, and analyzing the resulting outcomes, without consuming physical materials or machine time. This approach supports safe, repeatable practice and bridges the gap between conceptual knowledge and procedural expertise.

Following each simulation, CALLME guides learners through self-assessment and reflection tasks. These exercises reinforce cognitive retention and promote awareness by prompting learners to articulate the relationships between parameter changes and process results. CALLME's adaptive analytics engine continuously records and interprets interaction data, including task sequences, time on task, frequency of parameter adjustments, and error-correction patterns. This data is processed into learning vectors, which are then used to personalize the educational trajectory of each user.

Pedagogically, the platform is grounded in constructivist and experiential learning methods. Learners build understanding through direct interaction, reflection, and feedback, transforming passive content consumption into active knowledge construction. CALLME's architecture aligns with the principles of Industry 5.0, emphasizing personalization, human–machine collaboration, and data-informed decision-making in education.

Through this integration, VR simulations cease to be isolated visualization tools and instead become components of an intelligent, adaptive learning ecosystem. CALLME connects digital twin technology, analytics, and pedagogy within a single framework, enabling continuous improvement of both learner performance and curriculum design. The result is a holistic educational infrastructure that cultivates not only technical proficiency but also reflective, self-regulated learning behavior essential for future professionals in biomedical and engineering domains [13, 14].

4 Discussion

This integration of A-Frame and CALLME provides a practical blueprint for next-generation engineering and biomedical education. It combines visual immersion with AI-supported adaptivity, creating a data-rich environment for learners and instructors. The system is open-source, lightweight, and browser-based, suitable for classrooms, remote settings, and hybrid models. Pedagogically, it reflects constructivist and experiential principles: learners experiment, observe consequences, and reflect on dynamics. Research potential of this approach is based on the analyses of learning behavior, process understanding, and digital-twin interaction. On the other hand, the challenges can be defined with a need to: improving physics realism, sustain frame rate with complex meshes, and align analytics with outcomes. Although the proposed framework is conceptual, it enables demonstrative validation through learning analytics. Unlike traditional AM education, which relies primarily on static instruction and summative assessment, the presented system captures continuous interaction data such as parameter changes, time on task, and error-correction patterns. These behavioral indicators allow instructors to objectively assess how learners explore process variables and develop procedural understanding. Compared to conventional CAD-based or video-based instruction, the framework provides immediate visual feedback and adaptive task progression, supporting deeper conceptual learning and self-regulated experimentation. Future work will focus on collaborative multi-user modes, real-time printer synchronization, and advanced process visualization.

5 Conclusion

This paper presented a process-oriented educational framework that integrates browser-based VR simulation using A-Frame WebXR with the CALLME AI-supported learning platform for additive manufacturing education in medical engineering. By embedding the complete AM workflow—model preparation, parameter selection, fabrication, and defect analysis—into a single immersive environment, the proposed approach supports holistic understanding of process dependencies rather than isolated task execution.

The main contribution of this work lies in the structured coupling of immersive visualization with learning analytics. Unlike conventional AM education approaches that rely on static demonstrations or post-hoc assessments, the proposed framework enables continuous observation of learner behavior, parameter exploration, and decision-making strategies through real-time interaction data. By aligning immersive simulation with digital twin concepts, the framework supports a process-oriented understanding of additive manufacturing systems that extends beyond isolated task execution [16]. This process-oriented perspective aligns with constructivist learning principles and the human-centric vision of Industry 5.0, emphasizing personalization, transparency, and active learner engagement.

Although the framework is conceptual, it establishes a demonstrative foundation for educational validation by enabling objective analysis of learning processes through behavioral metrics such as time on task, interaction sequences, and error-correction patterns. These indicators provide a basis for future comparative studies with traditional instructional methods.

Future work will focus on empirical validation through controlled educational studies, expansion toward multi-material and metal AM processes, and the integration of collaborative multi-user VR scenarios. In the long term, the framework has the potential to evolve into a comprehensive digital twin–based educational ecosystem that bridges design, simulation, and manufacturing within medical and biomedical engineering curricula.

Acknowledgments. This research was supported by the ERASMUS+ Partnerships for cooperation and exchanges of practices (KA220) - "Biomedical Innovations through Digital Transformation of Additive Technologies and Knowledge Exchange - BIOMEDIX" - Project No. 2024-1-LV01-KA220- HED-000255929, "Extended Reality for Machine Tool Training" – XMAN (Project Reference: 2023-1-PL01-KA220-VET-000162134) and "CALLME" - Collaborative e-platform for innovation and educational enhancement in medical engineering, Funded by the European Union, ERASMUS+, 2022-2025, https://project-callme.eu/, 2022-1-RO01-KA220-HED-000087703.

References

1. Salmi M (2021) Additive manufacturing processes in medical applications. Materials 14(1):191. https://doi.org/10.3390/ma14010191
2. Gibson I, Rosen DW, Stucker B, Khorasani M (2021) Additive manufacturing technologies, 3rd edn. Springer, Cham. https://doi.org/10.1007/978-3-030-56127-7
3. Campbell I, Bourell D, Gibson I (2012) Additive manufacturing: rapid prototyping comes of age. Rapid Prototyp J 18(4):255–258. https://doi.org/10.1108/13552541211231563
4. Ford S, Despeisse M (2016) Additive manufacturing and sustainability: an exploratory study of environmental impacts and educational implications. J Clean Prod 137:1573–1587. https://doi.org/10.1016/j.jclepro.2016.04.150

5. Vitković N et al (2018) Software framework for the creation and application of personalized bone and plate implant geometrical models. J Healthcare Eng 2018:6025935. https://doi.org/10.1155/2018/6025935
6. A-Frame WebXR Documentation. https://aframe.io/docs/. Accessed 3 Nov 2025
7. European Commission (2020) Industry 5.0 – towards a sustainable, human-centric and resilient European industry. Publications Office of the European Union, Brussels. https://doi.org/10.2777/308407
8. Rengier F et al (2010) 3D printing based on imaging data: review of medical applications. Int J Comput. Assist Radiol Surg 5(4):335–341. https://doi.org/10.1007/s11548-010-0476-x
9. Moro C, Štromberga Z, Raikos A, Stirling A (2017) The effectiveness of virtual and augmented reality in health sciences and medical anatomy. Anat Sci Educ 10(6):549–559. https://doi.org/10.1002/ase.1696
10. Makransky G, Petersen GB (2019) Immersive virtual reality and learning: a meta-analysis. Educ Psychol Rev 31:775–799. https://doi.org/10.1007/s10648-019-09497-9
11. Radianti J, Majchrzak TA, Fromm J, Wohlgenannt I (2020) A systematic review of immersive virtual reality applications for higher education. Educ Inf Technol 25:495–519. https://doi.org/10.1007/s10639-019-09922-1
12. Fan H, Zhang H, Ma C, Wu T, Fuh JYH, Li B (2024) Enhancing metal additive manufacturing training with an advanced vision-language model: a pathway to immersive AR training for non-experts. J Manuf Syst 75:257–269. https://doi.org/10.1016/j.jmsy.2024.06.007
13. Tang YM, Chau KY, Kwok APK, Zhu T, Ma X (2022) A systematic review of immersive technology applications for medical practice and education. Educ Res Rev 35:100429. https://doi.org/10.1016/j.edurev.2021.100429
14. Yun YH, Shin DH, Choi HJ (2024) Perspectives of medical students and developers regarding virtual reality, augmented reality, mixed reality, and 3D printing technologies: survey study. JMIR XR and Spatial Computing 10(1):e54230. https://doi.org/10.2196/54230
15. de Visser H, Watson MO, Salvado O, Passenger JD (2011) Progress in virtual-reality simulators for surgical training and certification. Surg Endosc 25(7):2131–2139. https://doi.org/10.5694/j.1326-5377.2011.tb02942.x
16. Tene T, Garcia NB, Fiallos DC, Borja M, Gomez CV (2024) A systematic review of immersive educational technologies in medical physics and radiation physics. Front Med 11:1384799. https://doi.org/10.3389/fmed.2024.1384799

Parametric Optimization of Additively Manufactured Proximal Humerus Cloverleaf Plates Using the Method of Anatomical Features (MAF)

Nikola Vitković(✉), Aleksandar Trajkovic, Jovan Arandjelovic, Rajko Turudija, and Milica Barac

Faculty of Mechanical Engineering, University of Nis, Niš, Serbia
nikola.vitkovic@masfak.ni.ac.rs

Abstract. This paper presents a parametric modeling framework for the design and additive manufacturing (AM) of personalized fixation plates based on the Method of Anatomical Features (MAF). The study focuses on the proximal humerus cloverleaf plate-a complex, multi-branch construct for fracture stabilization-and demonstrates its adaptation to a low-cost polymer prototype fabricated by fused-deposition modeling (FDM). The proposed method defines a hierarchical feature structure in which key geometric parameters-curvature, plate thickness, branch orientation, and screw-hole pattern-are derived from anatomical descriptors obtained directly from patient-specific data. The MAF framework ensures consistent anatomical alignment and scalability of the design across individual morphologies. The workflow further demonstrates cross-anatomical reusability through a tibial adaptation case, showing that identical parametric logic can be transferred to other long bones by redefining landmark sets. The resulting approach enables efficient design iteration, manufacturability evaluation, and physical validation through AM prototypes.

Keywords: Parametric modeling · Additive manufacturing · Cloverleaf plate · Bone · MAF

1 Introduction

Personalized orthopedic implants play a crucial role in improving clinical outcomes in trauma and reconstructive surgery. Conventional fixation plates are typically designed according to averaged anatomical geometries, which often necessitates extensive intraoperative bending to achieve acceptable bone conformity. Such adjustments increase surgical time, introduce variability in implant positioning, and may compromise the mechanical performance and fatigue life of the fixation system. The increasing availability of high-resolution medical imaging, advanced computer-aided design (CAD), and AM technologies has enabled the development of patient-specific implants that better match individual anatomy and reduce the need for intraoperative modification.

F. Górski et al. (Eds.): MANUFACTURING 2026, LNME, pp. 12–23, 2026.
https://doi.org/10.1007/978-3-032-23089-8_2

Despite these technological advances, establishing a robust and reproducible digital workflow that links anatomical information, parametric modeling, and manufacturability evaluation remains a major challenge. Many existing approaches rely on direct surface morphing or manual remodeling of implant geometries, which limits scalability and introduces operator-dependent variability. Statistical shape modeling has been widely used to describe anatomical variability across populations; however, such models often lack direct control over functional implant features such as plate curvature continuity, screw-hole orientation, and segment topology [1]. Similarly, template-based design strategies offer rapid generation of patient-adapted plates but frequently sacrifice precise anatomical alignment and biomechanical intent during geometric warping [2]. In recent years, knowledge-based and feature-semantic modeling approaches have gained increasing attention in biomedical CAD, as they enable explicit embedding of anatomical and functional information directly into the design structure. Parametric implant models driven by anatomical descriptors have been shown to significantly improve design consistency while preserving essential biomechanical relationships between implant features and the underlying bone geometry [3, 4]. When combined with additive manufacturing, such approaches allow rapid iteration, direct manufacturability assessment, and efficient physical validation of implant concepts.

Additive manufacturing has evolved from a rapid-prototyping technology to a viable production route for medical devices, including load-bearing orthopedic implants. Advances in process control, material qualification, and international standards have facilitated the clinical adoption of additively manufactured implants, while design-for-additive-manufacturing (DfAM) principles increasingly influence implant geometry, thickness distribution, and support-free design strategies [5, 6]. However, many generative and optimization-based design frameworks struggle to maintain strict anatomical correspondence and clinically acceptable screw trajectories, which are essential requirements for fixation plate applications.

MAF addresses these limitations by providing a structured framework for extracting invariant anatomical landmarks and embedding them into a parametric CAD model. By defining a hierarchy of reference geometrical entities derived from bone morphology, MAF enables automatic adaptation of implant geometry while preserving functional relationships such as curvature logic, segment orientation, and screw-hole alignment [7]. In this study, the MAF-driven parametric approach is applied to the design of a proximal humerus cloverleaf plate, selected due to its complex three-dimensional curvature and clinical relevance in upper-limb fracture fixation. Furthermore, the same parametric logic is extended to a tibial case to demonstrate cross-anatomical reusability and the general applicability of the proposed framework.

2 Background and Motivation

Statistical Shape Modeling (SSM) techniques describe anatomical variability using population-based datasets and principal component analysis, allowing efficient representation of morphological trends. Nevertheless, SSM-based approaches usually provide limited control over functionally critical implant features such as screw-hole orientation, curvature continuity, or localized thickness variation, which are essential for fixation plate performance [8]. Template-based design strategies attempt to overcome this limitation by warping predefined implant geometries to patient anatomy, enabling faster design generation but often at the expense of precise anatomical alignment and biomechanical intent [9].

In parallel, recent advances in deep learning–based surface reconstruction and implicit anatomical representation have significantly improved the accuracy of digital bone models derived from medical imaging data [10, 11]. Despite these advances, most data-driven pipelines focus primarily on geometry reconstruction, while the translation of reconstructed anatomy into a fully functional, manufacturable implant remains largely dependent on manual modeling and expert intervention.

From an engineering design perspective, generative design and topology optimization frameworks introduce parameterized search spaces capable of exploring numerous geometric alternatives under mechanical constraints. Although such methods are effective for lightweight structural components, their direct application to orthopedic fixation plates is constrained by the need to preserve strict anatomical correspondence, clinically acceptable screw trajectories, and surgical accessibility, which are difficult to encode solely through optimization objectives [12].

The Method of Anatomical Features (MAF) addresses these challenges by establishing a structured link between anatomical intelligence and engineering parameterization. By identifying invariant morphological landmarks—such as curvature extremes, functional ridges, and anatomical axes MAF enables the creation of parametric models in which implant geometry adapts automatically to individual anatomy while preserving functional relationships [7, 13]. This feature-based paradigm differs fundamentally from purely geometric fitting approaches, as it explicitly retains design intent and biomechanical logic throughout the adaptation process.

In parallel, additive manufacturing technologies have matured from rapid prototyping tools into clinically validated production methods for orthopedic implants. The increasing adoption of DfAM principles has emphasized manufacturability-aware geometry definition, including overhang limitations, minimum wall thickness, and support minimization [14, 15]. Embedding such constraints directly within a parametric implant model allows real-time feedback on manufacturability during geometric adaptation, rather than as a post-design validation step.

The combination of MAF-driven feature extraction and AM-oriented parametric design represents a new class of feature-semantic modeling where geometry, anatomy, and manufacturing constraints coexist in a unified model. This research adopts that paradigm for the complex proximal-humerus cloverleaf plate, extending it toward cross-anatomical reuse on the tibia to illustrate the generality of the method.

3 Methodology

The developed workflow integrates anatomical data acquisition, feature-driven parametric modeling, and additive manufacturing preparation into a unified digital framework for patient-specific fixation plate design. All geometric parameters are explicitly linked to anatomically defined landmarks using the MAF method, ensuring reproducibility, traceability, and anatomical consistency across subjects.

3.1 Anatomical Data and Reverse Modeling

Two computed tomography (CT) scans of the left humerus were used in this study, acquired using a Toshiba 64-slice scanner under a standard clinical protocol (slice thickness $\leq$ 1 mm, in accordance with recommended resolution for orthopedic implant design) [16]. A polygonal surface model was generated from the volumetric data and imported into CATIA V5 for reverse engineering. Mesh filtering and repair operations were performed to reduce segmentation noise while preserving cortical geometry, followed by surface reconstruction using spline sections positioned in anatomically meaningful planes.

The reconstruction followed the principles of the Method of Anatomical Features (MAF), with explicitly defined Referential Geometrical Entities (RGEs). These included characteristic points, axes, and planes: the Z-axis corresponding to the metaphyseal–shaft axis, the X-axis defined through the projection of distal epicondyles, and the Y-axis orthogonal to the X–Z plane. Anatomical imaging planes—anteroposterior (AP), lateromedial (LM), and axial—were used as reference planes for section placement and geometric reconstruction. Separate surface patches were generated for the proximal, shaft, and distal regions and merged into a continuous humerus surface model.

The accuracy of anatomical landmark extraction depends on CT image resolution, segmentation strategy, and operator-dependent placement of reconstruction splines. Variability in epicondylar landmark identification and metaphyseal axis estimation may introduce geometric deviations on the order of 0.5–1.0 mm, which is consistent with previously reported uncertainties in CT-based bone modeling workflows [17, 18]. These uncertainties were considered acceptable for fixation plate design, as they remain below clinically relevant tolerance thresholds.

3.2 Parametric Definition of the Modified Cloverleaf Plate

The fixation plate was defined as a feature-parametric solid whose geometry adapts to humeral morphology while preserving topological consistency. Primary dimensional parameters were measured in the AP plane of the reconstructed humerus model and included:

- RPmax – maximal proximal radius to the anatomical axis (proximal head envelope),
- RDmax – maximal distal radius to the anatomical axis,
- Mwidth – chord-based radius controlling proximal head wrapping.

These parameters were selected to capture the dominant curvature and width variations of the proximal humerus while limiting the total number of degrees of freedom, thereby improving robustness and repeatability of the automated design process [19].

A uniform plate thickness of 2.0 mm was applied to generate the solid implant geometry. This value was selected based on reported clinical fixation plate designs for the proximal humerus, where thickness values between 2.0 and 3.5 mm are commonly adopted to balance bending stiffness, fatigue resistance, and soft-tissue compatibility [20, 21]. The chosen thickness prioritizes anatomical conformity and reduced implant prominence, which is particularly relevant in minimally invasive fixation scenarios.

Curvature limits were implicitly controlled through RPmax and RDmax to prevent excessive plate bending that could compromise manufacturability or induce high residual stresses. Acceptable geometrical fit deviations were preliminarily constrained to below 2.5 mm, reflecting reported tolerances for pre-contoured anatomical plates and accounting for the presence of periosteal tissue and intraoperative plate adaptation [22, 23].

To achieve proper anatomical seating, two rigid-body adjustments were introduced: a lateral–medial angle (LMA) rotation about the plate axis and a transverse angle (TA) rotation about an axis located distal to the metaphysis. In the evaluated configuration, the LMA was approximately 11°, while the TA was approximately 0.5°. A final normal translation of 1 mm from the LM plane was applied to prevent initial surface interpenetration and to reflect standard implant–bone spacing reported in orthopedic fixation practice [24].

3.3 Geometrical Fit Evaluation

Geometrical fit was evaluated by comparing intersections of the plate and bone surfaces within the AP plane. Deviations were quantified as normal distances between corresponding intersection splines. The maximum deviation in the proximal epiphysis was 2.27 mm, while the maximum deviation in the proximal diaphysis was 2.44 mm. Approximately 70% of the plate contact surface exhibited deviations below 0.5 mm, indicating satisfactory anatomical conformity.

The accuracy of the reconstructed humerus surface relative to the original polygonal model showed typical deviations between 0.4 and 0.8 mm, which are within the accuracy range reported for CT-based reverse-engineered bone models used in orthopedic implant design [17, 18].

To preliminarily assess functional performance, the generated plate geometry was evaluated under a simplified load-case assumption representative of proximal humerus fixation, considering axial compression and bending moments induced by arm weight and muscle forces. While full finite element simulations are beyond the scope of the present study, the continuous curvature and absence of sharp geometric discontinuities are expected to promote favorable stress distribution and reduced stress concentrations compared to manually contoured or template-based designs [23, 24].

Unlike template-based or morphing-based plate adaptation methods, which rely on predefined reference geometries or mesh deformation techniques, the proposed framework derives plate geometry directly from anatomically defined features. This reduces sensitivity to mesh quality, improves interpretability of design parameters, and enables transparent control over clinically relevant geometric constraints [19, 23] (Fig. 1).

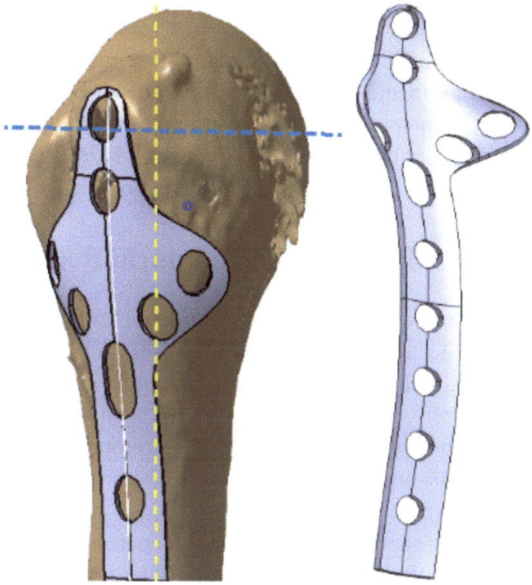

Fig. 1. Personalized cloverleaf type internal plate model

4 Additive-Manufacturing Prototype

A fused deposition modeling (FDM) process was employed for the rapid and cost-effective validation of the designed implant geometry, enabling physical inspection of anatomical conformity prior to metallic additive manufacturing. The prototype was fabricated using a desktop FDM printer equipped with a 0.4 mm brass nozzle and 1.75 mm polylactic acid (PLA) filament. Printing parameters were selected based on preliminary trials to ensure dimensional stability and adequate surface quality. A layer height of 0.15 mm, three perimeter walls, five top and bottom layers, and a gyroid infill density of 60% were applied. A printing temperature of 210 °C and a bed temperature of 60 °C were used to ensure stable material deposition and sufficient bed adhesion.

The build orientation was defined with the concave anatomical surface facing upward to minimize the need for support structures and preserve curvature fidelity along the humeral contour. The total fabrication time for a single plate was approximately 2 h, including printer calibration and bed preparation. Following fabrication, minor support remnants were removed, and the contact surface was lightly polished using 600-grit abrasive paper to improve visual assessment of curvature continuity.

Dimensional accuracy was evaluated by comparing the printed prototype with the nominal CAD geometry using a 3D optical scan imported into CATIA V5. The measured dimensional deviation remained within ±0.4 mm, while the root-mean-square surface deviation was 0.28 mm. Such accuracy is sufficient for educational use, pre-surgical visualization, and early-stage design validation, as commonly reported for polymer-based AM prototypes in orthopedic applications [25].

From a manufacturing perspective, the successful fabrication confirmed that the integrated design-for-additive-manufacturing constraints—maximum overhang angle below 45°, minimum wall thickness above 1.2 mm, and minimum hole diameter of 3.5 mm—were correctly embedded within the parametric model. No structural defects, layer delamination, or significant surface artifacts were observed, indicating that the generated geometry can be manufactured without extensive support generation. These results establish a reliable foundation for subsequent validation using metallic additive manufacturing processes, such as laser powder bed fusion.

5 Parametric Reusability Across Anatomical Regions

Although the proposed framework was initially validated on the proximal humerus, its primary strength lies in the ability to transfer identical parametric logic to different skeletal regions while maintaining both anatomical conformity and engineering constraints. The feature hierarchy, variable naming structure, and dependency relationships remain unchanged, whereas only the anatomical descriptors defined by the Method of Anatomical Features (MAF) are replaced with those extracted from a new anatomical dataset.

This modular structure enables the creation of anatomically equivalent implant design procedures for multiple long bones, including the tibia, radius, and ulna, without rebuilding the CAD model from scratch. Once new landmark sets are defined, the governing parametric relationships automatically regenerate plate curvature, thickness distribution, and screw-hole orientation relative to the new anatomical reference frame. As a result, the same CAD procedure effectively functions as a morphological generator that adapts implant geometry to any bone characterized by MAF descriptors.

The transformation procedure involves constructing a local anatomical coordinate system specific to the target bone. For the humerus, this system is defined by the humeral head center, the greater tuberosity apex, and the shaft axis, whereas for the tibia it is defined by the medial plateau centroid, the anterior crest apex, and the diaphyseal axis. Affine transformations between these coordinate systems allow all dependent geometric entities—plate segments, curvature profiles, and screw trajectories—to be recomputed automatically. Similar cross-anatomical reuse strategies have been reported as a key advantage of knowledge-based and feature-driven implant design frameworks, particularly for reducing modeling time and improving design consistency [26].

Transformation of Anatomical Reference Frames

In the humerus, the local coordinate frame is defined by the humeral-head center C_1, the greater-tuberosity apex C_2, and the shaft axis (A_1–A_2). For the tibia, the transformation involves identifying:

- the medial-plateau centroid C_1',
- the anterior-crest apex C_2', and
- the longitudinal diaphyseal axis (A_1'–A_2').

These landmarks define a tibia-specific anatomical reference frame $\{x', y', z'\}$, which replaces the humeral coordinate system during geometric regeneration. All higher-level parametric relations, including segment vectors, curvature-mapping functions, and screw-hole orientation matrices, are automatically recomputed relative to the new coordinate system using affine transformations. Parametric adaptation of the proximal-humerus cloverleaf plate is shown in Fig. 2.

This transformation strategy preserves the hierarchical dependency structure of the parametric model. Screw-hole trajectories remain orthogonal to local surface normals, while curvature continuity and edge-fillet propagation are governed by the same underlying parametric relationships. Similar coordinate-based anatomical transformation strategies have been reported as effective mechanisms for enabling reusable implant design workflows across multiple skeletal regions [27].

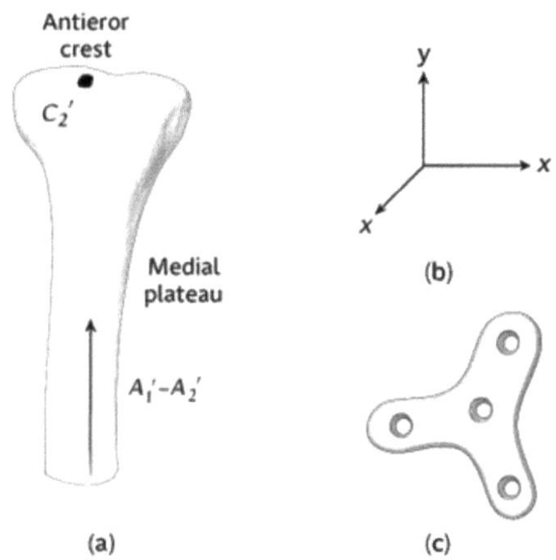

Fig. 2. – Parametric adaptation of the proximal-humerus cloverleaf plate to tibial geometry. (a) Extraction of tibial anatomical landmarks using the Method of Anatomical Features (MAF): medial plateau centroid ($C_1{}'$), anterior crest apex ($C_2{}'$), and diaphyseal axis ($A_1{}'$–$A_2{}'$). (b) Affine transformation between the humeral anatomical reference frame $\{x^m, y^m, z^m\}$ and the tibial reference frame $\{x'^m, y'^m, z'^m\}$. (c) Automatically regenerated bi-lobe tibial plate geometry, preserving parametric dependency structure, curvature continuity, and screw-hole orientation rules defined in the original humeral design.

5.1 Geometric and Structural Adaptation

The tibial morphology differs significantly from that of the humerus. While the proximal humerus exhibits a rounded, multi-axial curvature to accommodate the rotator cuff, the proximal tibia features an elongated and flatter cortical surface dominated by compressive rather than torsional loads. Accordingly, the design kernel adjusts several geometric variables:

- Curvature radius R decreases from 45–60 mm to 25–35 mm to match the medial plateau curvature.
- Branch angle θ is reduced from 120° (three-lobe configuration) to 70–90°, forming a bi-lobe plate that spans the metaphyseal flare.
- Plate thickness t increases to 3.0–3.5 mm to improve bending stiffness under axial load.
- Screw orientation α is modified toward 90°, providing nearly perpendicular trajectories to the cortical surface for axial compression.

Summary of key parameters for humeral and tibial plate adaptations is given in the Table 1.

Table 1. Summary of key geometric and manufacturing parameters for humeral and tibial plate adaptations

Parameter	Proximal humerus	Proximal tibia
Curvature radius R (mm)	45–60	25–35
Branch angle θ (deg)	~120 (tri-lobe)	70–90 (bi-lobe)
Plate thickness t (mm)	2.0	3.0–3.5
Max geometric deviation (mm)	2.44	$\leq$ 2.5
RMS surface deviation (mm)	0.6–0.9	0.7–1.0
Overhang area < 45° (%)	94%	92%
CAD regeneration time	< 2 min	< 2 min

Because all geometric parameters are functionally linked within the parametric model, these updates propagate automatically through dependent relationships, including offset distance $\delta(u, v)$, segment blending radius r_f, and taper ratio τ. This ensures consistent topology, curvature continuity, and manufacturability without the need for manual remodeling. Comparable parameter-driven adaptation strategies have been highlighted as a key advantage of feature-based implant design in recent orthopedic CAD studies [28].

5.2 Manufacturing Evaluation

From a manufacturing perspective, both polymer-based FDM and metallic powder-bed fusion processes can be accommodated within the same parametric framework. For the tibial variant, identical slicing parameters and mesh resolutions were retained, with only a minor orientation adjustment of approximately 20° about the longitudinal axis to reduce support requirements. Overhang analysis confirmed that more than 92% of the surface exhibited angles below 45°, satisfying common design-for-additive-manufacturing (DfAM) criteria and enabling efficient post-processing.

Because the underlying feature hierarchy and dependency structure remain unchanged, design validation and manufacturing simulation steps can be automated across different implant variants. This consistency simplifies manufacturability assessment and reduces the need for repeated manual verification when adapting the design to new anatomical regions. Similar automation benefits have been reported in recent studies focusing on parametric and knowledge-based implant manufacturing workflows [29].

6 Clinical and Educational Implications

From a practical perspective, the presented results demonstrate that the proposed parametric framework enables anatomically conforming implant designs while maintaining manufacturability constraints across different skeletal regions. Automatic regeneration of geometry without manual remodeling significantly reduces design time, while consistent curvature and thickness control support reliable additive manufacturing. These characteristics indicate strong potential for scalable patient-specific implant libraries and streamlined clinical workflows.

In addition to clinical applications, the developed framework offers significant educational value. The additively manufactured prototypes provide tangible representations of the relationship between anatomical landmarks, parametric equations, and manufacturing constraints, making them suitable for teaching biomedical engineering students and clinicians. Similar applications of physical AM models for education and preoperative planning have been shown to improve anatomical understanding and interdisciplinary communication.

7 Discussion

The presented results demonstrate that MAF-based feature modeling effectively embeds anatomical knowledge within the parametric design structure, enabling automated adaptation of fixation plate geometry to patient-specific bone morphology. Unlike purely geometric morphing or statistical approaches, the proposed method preserves functional design intent, including curvature logic, screw-hole trajectories, and segment topology, across different anatomical variants.

This cross-anatomical reusability is critical for the development of next-generation implant libraries. A single validated parametric workflow can be employed to generate families of fixation plates directly from patient-specific imaging data, significantly reducing design effort and supporting standardized manufacturing and validation procedures.

The integration of design-for-additive-manufacturing constraints directly within the CAD model ensures that generated implant geometries are immediately manufacturable without extensive post-design modification. The successful fabrication and dimensional validation of the FDM prototype confirm that the parametric definitions and embedded constraints produce geometries suitable for physical realization. Moreover, the extension of the same parametric logic to the tibial case highlights the efficiency and robustness of the proposed framework, as complex geometric adaptations are achieved without manual remodeling.

Compared with optimization-driven design approaches, which often struggle to maintain strict anatomical correspondence, the MAF-driven method provides explicit control over clinically relevant features. This balance between anatomical fidelity, engineering control, and manufacturability is increasingly recognized as a critical requirement for patient-specific orthopedic implant design.

Despite these advantages, certain limitations should be acknowledged. The present study focuses on geometric conformity and manufacturability, while experimental biomechanical testing and in vivo validation were beyond its scope. Future work will therefore focus on metallic additive manufacturing, mechanical testing, and automated anatomical landmark detection to further enhance the robustness and clinical applicability of the framework.

8 Conclusions

A feature-based parametric design framework for the development of personalized proximal humerus cloverleaf plates was presented using the Method of Anatomical Features (MAF). The proposed workflow enables automatic generation of patient-specific implant geometries by directly linking anatomical landmarks to parametric design variables, thereby preserving functional relationships and design intent.

The successful fabrication and evaluation of a polymer-based additive manufacturing prototype confirmed the feasibility of the approach for rapid design validation and educational use. Furthermore, the demonstrated transfer of the same parametric logic to a tibial case highlights the cross-anatomical reusability of the framework and its potential for generating implant families across multiple skeletal regions.

By integrating anatomical intelligence, parametric modeling, and manufacturability constraints within a unified CAD environment, the proposed methodology contributes to the development of intelligent and reconfigurable biomedical manufacturing systems. Future work will focus on metallic additive manufacturing validation, mechanical testing, and further automation of anatomical feature extraction to support clinical translation.

Acknowledgements. This research was supported by the ERASMUS+ Partnerships for cooperation and exchanges of practices (KA220) - "Biomedical Innovations through Digital Transformation of Additive Technologies and Knowledge Exchange - BIOMEDIX" - Project No. 2024-1-LV01-KA220- HED-000255929 and "Extended Reality for Machine Tool Training" – XMAN (Project Reference: 2023-1-PL01-KA220-VET-000162134).

References

1. Rashid MM et al (2017) Geometrical model creation methods for human humerus bone and modified cloverleaf plate. J Sci Ind Res 76(10):631–639
2. Stojković M et al (2018) Reverse modelling of human long bones using T-splines – case of tibia. Tehnički vjesnik 25(6):1753–1760. https://doi.org/10.17559/TV-20180129210021
3. Vitković N, Radović L, Trajanović M, Manić M (2019) 3D point cloud model of human bio form created by the application of geometric morphometrics and method of anatomical features: human tibia example. Filomat 33(4):1217–1225. https://doi.org/10.2298/FIL1904217V
4. Ambellan F, Tack A, Ehlke M, Zachow S (2019) Statistical shape models: understanding and mastering variation in anatomy. In: Biomedical image analysis. Springer, Cham, pp 67–84. https://doi.org/10.1007/978-3-030-19385-0_5
5. Mao Z, Yang M, Chen X, Shao J (2021) An integrated computer-aided approach for parametric investigation of anatomic plate design. Virtual Phys Prototyp 16(3):282–295. https://doi.org/10.1080/13102818.2021.1922094

6. National center for advancing translational sciences (2020) 3D print exchange. NIH NCATS
7. ISO/ASTM 52900 (2021) Additive manufacturing — general principles — fundamentals and vocabulary. ISO/ASTM
8. Gibson I, Rosen DW, Stucker B, Khorasani M (2021) Additive Manufacturing Technologies, 3rd edn. Springer. https://doi.org/10.1007/978-3-030-56127-7
9. Campbell I, Bourell D, Gibson I (2012) Additive manufacturing: rapid prototyping comes of age. Rapid Prototyp J 18(4):255–258. https://doi.org/10.1108/13552541211231563
10. Wong KC (2016) 3D-printed patient-specific applications in orthopedics. Orthop Res Rev 8:57–66. https://doi.org/10.2147/ORR.S99653
11. ASTM F3303–18 (2018) Standard specification for Ti-6Al-4V (ELI) powder for additive manufacturing processes. ASTM International
12. Vitković N, Manić M, Trajanović M, Mitković M, Arsić S, Stojković M (2016) The reverse engineering of human organs based on the application of method of anatomical features. Tehnički vjesnik 23(4):1173–1180. https://doi.org/10.17559/TV-20160201081147
13. Vitković N, Stojković JR, Korunović N et al (2023) Extra-articular distal Humerus plate 3D model creation by using the method of anatomical features. Materials 16(15):5409. https://doi.org/10.3390/ma16155409
14. Moosabeiki V et al (2023) 3D printed patient-specific fixation plates. J Mech Behav Biomed Mater 148:106173. https://doi.org/10.1016/j.jmbbm.2023.106173
15. Maintz M et al (2024) Patient-specific implants made of 3D printed bioresorbable polymers. 3D Printing in Medicine 10(1):13. https://doi.org/10.1186/s41205-024-00207-0
16. Van den Broeck J, Vereecke E, Vander SJ (2014) Segmentation accuracy of long bones. Med Eng Phys 36(7):949–956. https://doi.org/10.1016/j.medengphy.2014.03.016
17. van Eijnatten M, van Dijk R, Dobbe J, Streekstra GJ, Koivisto J, Wolff J (2018) CT image segmentation methods for bone used in medical additive manufacturing. Med Eng Phys 51:6–16. https://doi.org/10.1016/j.medengphy.2017.10.008
18. Gardner MJ et al (2007) The importance of medial support in locked plating of proximal humerus fractures. J Orthop Trauma 21(3):185–191. https://doi.org/10.1097/BOT.0b013e3180333094
19. Südkamp N et al (2009) Open reduction and internal fixation of proximal humeral fractures. J Bone Joint Surgery (Am) 91(6):1320–1328. https://doi.org/10.2106/JBJS.H.00006
20. Schmutz B et al (2008) Fit assessment of anatomic plates for the distal medial tibia. J Orthop Trauma 22(4):258–263. https://doi.org/10.1097/BOT.0b013e31816b10ba
21. Harith H et al (2016) Can we safely deform a plate to fit every bone? Med Eng Phys 38(4):357–364. https://doi.org/10.1016/j.medengphy.2015.11.012
22. Miller DL, Goswami T (2007) A review of locking compression plate biomechanics. Clin Biomech 22(10):1049–1062. https://doi.org/10.1016/j.clinbiomech.2007.08.004
23. Park S M et al (2021) Design process of patient-specific osteosynthesis plates using topology optimization. J Comput Design Eng 8(4):1095–1107. https://doi.org/10.1093/jcde/qwab047
24. Wang L, Guo KJ, He KJ, Zhu H (2021) Bone morphological feature extraction for customized bone plate design. Sci Rep 11:16543. https://doi.org/10.1038/s41598-021-94924-9
25. Aranđelović J, Vitković N, Korunović N (2024) A methodology for personalization of Humerus shaft plate. AIP Conf Proc 3125:030011. https://doi.org/10.1063/5.0216396
26. Neamah ZH (2024) Custom design of fracture fixation plates. AIP Conf Proc 3232:040002
27. Kanagalingam S et al (2023) Detailed design for additive manufacturing of high tibial osteotomy plates. Prog Addit Manuf 8:409–426. https://doi.org/10.1007/s40964-022-00342-2
28. Mobarak MH et al (2023) Recent advances of additive manufacturing in implant fabrication. Appl Surf Sci Adv 18:100462. https://doi.org/10.1016/j.apsadv.2023.100462
29. Murugan S, Vinodh S (2024) Holistic review on design for additive manufacturing. Prog Addit Manuf 10(8):4497–4532. https://doi.org/10.1007/s40964-024-00887-4

MAF-Based Workflow for Parametric Modeling of Anatomical Surfaces Using NURBS and SubD

Diana Elena Horincar[1], Răzvan Păcurar[1], Petru Berce[1], Nikola Vitković[2], Sanja Stojanović[3], and Monica Rău[1](✉)

[1] Technical University of Cluj-Napoca, Cluj-Napoca, Romania
Monica.Rau@campus.utcluj.ro
[2] Faculty of Mechanical Engineering, University of Niš, Niš, Serbia
[3] Faculty of Medicine, University of Niš, Niš, Serbia

Abstract. Chronic wounds require accurate morphological characterization and personalized therapeutic devices that conform to patient-specific anatomy. This work presents a parametric modeling workflow based on the Method of Anatomical Features (MAF) for reconstructing anatomical wound surfaces using NURBS and Subdivision (SubD) representations. The pipeline combines deep-learning-based segmentation, curvature-driven MAF point extraction, parametric surface reconstruction, and surface offsetting for personalized cover generation. Experiments show sub-millimeter correspondence between original wound boundaries and reconstructed surfaces, with total processing times below ten seconds per case. We also detail NURBS parameterization, subdivision stopping criteria, and an adaptive MAF thresholding strategy to enhance reproducibility and compatibility with additive manufacturing.

Keywords: MAF · NURBS · SubD · Parametric modeling · Additive manufacturing · Personalized medicine · 3D reconstruction

1 Introduction

Chronic wounds represent a significant healthcare burden and require accurate morphological assessment to enable personalized therapeutic solutions. Deep-learning-based medical image analysis is now standard in this context [1, 2], and recent reviews on advanced wound dressings emphasize anatomically conforming, patient-specific devices [3, 4]. Although digital tools for wound management have advanced, the design of patient-specific covers and scaffolds often remains manual and inconsistent due to the lack of automated 3D modeling workflows capable of capturing individual anatomical geometry.

Existing reconstruction pipelines usually rely on dense triangulated meshes, which are visually accurate but difficult to parameterize, modify, or reuse over time. Mesh-based processing, repair, and scaffold design have been explored in several works [5–8], but these representations are not ideal for parametric manipulation or longitudinal adaptation.

F. Górski et al. (Eds.): MANUFACTURING 2026, LNME, pp. 24–31, 2026.
https://doi.org/10.1007/978-3-032-23089-8_3

The *Method of Anatomical Features* (MAF) provides a mathematical frame-work for extracting stable anatomical landmarks from biological structures and has been successfully applied to reverse engineering of bones and parametric modeling of organs [9–11]. By linking curvature-derived geometric descriptors with anatomical relevance, MAF enables reproducible, parametric surface reconstruction.

This study introduces a streamlined workflow that integrates MAF with parametric surface representations, specifically the Non-Uniform Rational B-Splines (NURBS) and Subdivision (SubD) surfaces—for reconstructing wound geometries and generating personalized covers suitable for additive manufacturing. The workflow spans segmentation, feature extraction, surface reconstruction, and parametric offsetting, focusing on clarity, reproducibility, and anatomical fidelity. For broader background on additive manufacturing technologies and terminology, we refer the reader to [12, 13].

The main contributions of this work are:

1. A MAF-based parametric modeling pipeline for generating personalized surface reconstructions using NURBS and SubD surfaces.
2. Integration of deep-learning-based wound segmentation with curvature-driven feature extraction.
3. Parametric surface offsetting for personalized wound or anatomical cover generation compatible with additive manufacturing.
4. Quantitative validation demonstrating sub-millimeter accuracy and near real-time processing performance.

2 Materials and Methods

2.1 Data Acquisition and Segmentation

High-resolution clinical images were captured under controlled lighting with a calibration marker of known size to ensure metric scaling. Segmentation of wound or anatomical regions was performed using the DeepSkin Convolutional Neural Network (CNN), trained for boundary detection and region classification. The DeepSkin CNN model was used as provided by the original authors; no additional retraining was performed in this study, and no separate train/test split was required. The binary mask $M(x, y) \in \{0, 1\}$ was processed using a marching squares algorithm to extract the wound boundary:

$$\{c_i\}_{i=1}^{N} = \mathrm{Boundary}(\mathrm{M(x, y)}). \tag{1}$$

Each pixel coordinate (x_i, y_i) was converted to metric space using the calibration factor s:

$$(X_i, Y_i) = s\ (x_i, y_i). \tag{2}$$

This produced a dense boundary curve representing the anatomical contour (segmentation and boundary extraction are illustrated in Fig. 1). However, the raw point cloud—often consisting of hundreds of points—was unsuitable for direct surface modeling and required feature-based reduction.

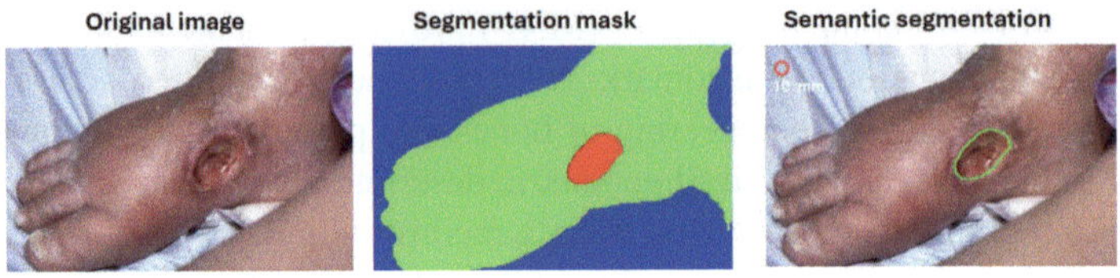

Fig. 1. Segmentation result and boundary extraction with calibration marker.

2.2 MAF Point Extraction

The Method of Anatomical Features (MAF) identifies geometrically and anatomically significant points along the boundary based on curvature extrema, as illustrated in Fig. 2.

Curvature $\kappa(s)$ along the contour is computed as:

$$k(s) = \frac{x\prime(s)y\prime\prime(s) - y\prime(s)x\prime\prime(s)}{\left(x\prime(s)^2 + y\prime(s)^2\right)^{3/2}} \tag{3}$$

The corresponding curvature plot is shown in Fig. 3.

The local maxima and minima correspond to corners, inflection points, or protrusions—features that often coincide with anatomical landmarks. To ensure reproducibility

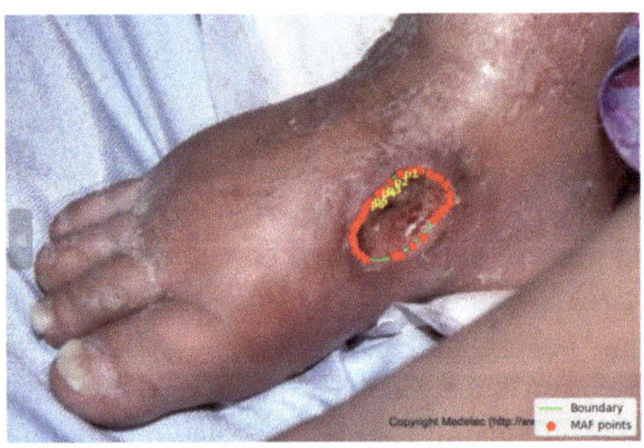

Fig. 2. Boundary with MAF points.

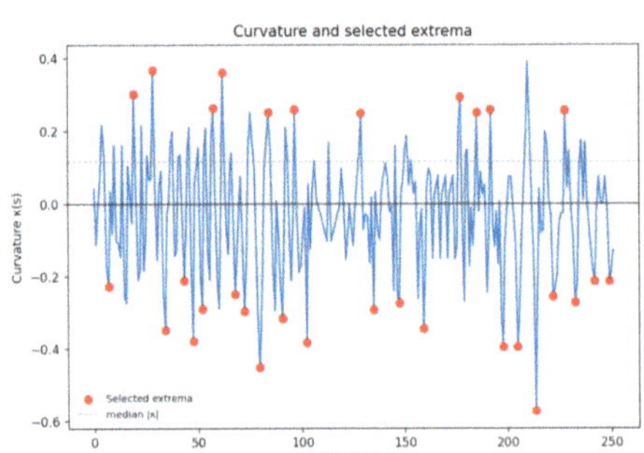

Fig. 3. Curvature plot along the segmented boundary.

and suppress noise, curvature extrema are filtered using an adaptive rule:

$$| K_i |> \alpha \cdot \overline{|K|}, \quad \alpha = 1.2, \tag{4}$$

where $|\kappa|$ is the mean absolute curvature along the contour. This removes minor fluctuations while preserving anatomically relevant landmarks. The resulting reduced set of MAF points is denoted $\{p_k\}_{k=1}^{M}$, where $M \ll N$. These MAF points serve as stable parametric anchors for subsequent surface modeling.

2.3 Surface Modeling Using NURBS and SubD

NURBS-Based Surface Generation. The surface is constructed using MAF points as control nodes. Boundary points form the outer control polygon, whereas interior points are generated along a MAF-based medial axis using curvature-weighted interpolation. The weights emphasize the maximum curvature to ensure conformance in critical anatomical regions.

NURBS Implementation Details. We employ standard CAD-based NURBS surfaces following the mathematical definitions implemented in the geomdl (NURBS-Python) library [14], which provides a widely used open-source implementation of the algorithms formalized in *The NURBS Book* [15]. In our workflow, MAF-derived points define the control structure of the surface, while the CAD kernel performs geometric interpolation.

We use degree $p = 3$ along the boundary direction and $q = 2$ along the medial direction, with clamped, non-uniform knot vectors in both parametric directions. The weights w_{ij} are automatically assigned by the CAD engine using curvature-based emphasis.

The resulting surface is defined as:

$$S(u, v) = \frac{\sum_{i=0}^{n} \sum_{j=0}^{m} N_{i,p}(u) M_{j,p}(v)\ w_{ij} P_{ij}}{\sum_{i=0}^{n} \sum_{j=0}^{m} N_{i,p}(u) M_{j,p}(v)\ w_{ij}} \tag{5}$$

where P_{ij} are control points, w_{ij} are weights, and $N_{i,p}$, $M_{j,q}$ are B-spline basis functions. A representative comparison between NURBS and SubD reconstructions is shown in Fig. 4.

Subdivision (SubD) Surface Generation. A constrained Delaunay triangulation defines connectivity, and the Catmull–Clark subdivision algorithm is applied iteratively until a smooth C^2-continuous surface is achieved [16]. For irregular or lobed geometries, SubD surfaces offer superior flexibility. Each MAF boundary point becomes a vertex in the SubD control mesh, with additional interior vertices placed along medial features.

In this work, the Catmull–Clark subdivision is applied for a fixed number of three iterations, chosen empirically because further refinement changes the surface by less than 0.1 mm in the RMS deviation. Using a fixed iteration count ensures consistent and reproducible behavior across all cases. The qualitative difference between NURBS and SubD reconstructions for a representative wound geometry is illustrated in Fig. 4.

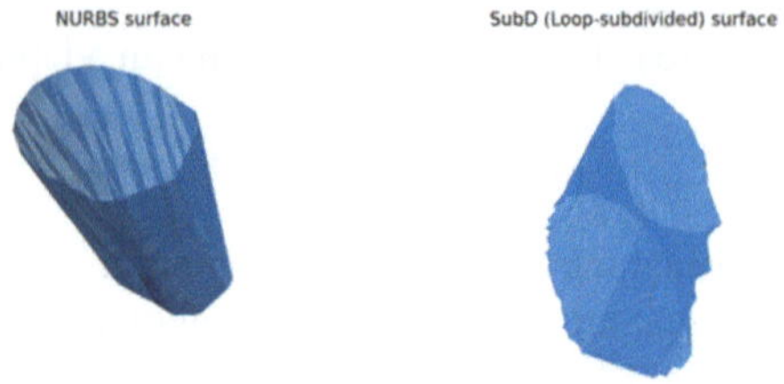

Fig. 4. Comparison of NURBS and SubD surface reconstructions for a curved wound geometry. Both models represent the full 3D anatomical surface; the cover is later obtained as a thin, flexible shell by normal offsetting this geometry, not by extruding a flat patch.

2.4 Wound or Anatomical Cover Generation

The surface $S(u, v)$ in (5) already parameterizes the *curved* anatomical region around the wound, including the surrounding skin. The cover is modeled as a thin, elastic shell that follows this 3D geometry and can be bent in vivo over the wound when fabricated in Nylon.

The shell is obtained by offsetting the reconstructed surface along its normal direction:

$$S_{offset}(u, v) = S(u, v) + t\,\mathbf{n}(u, v), \tag{6}$$

where t is the desired thickness of the cover (1–3 mm) and $\mathbf{n}(u, v)$ is the unit normal field. Thus, the offset operation only adds a controlled thickness in the normal (approximately Z) direction, while preserving the original 3D curvature of the anatomical surface. Edges are adaptively reinforced on the basis of local curvature. Ventilation and fluid channels are generated parametrically by projecting perforation patterns onto the surface. The complete workflow for personalized cover generation is summarized in Fig. 5.

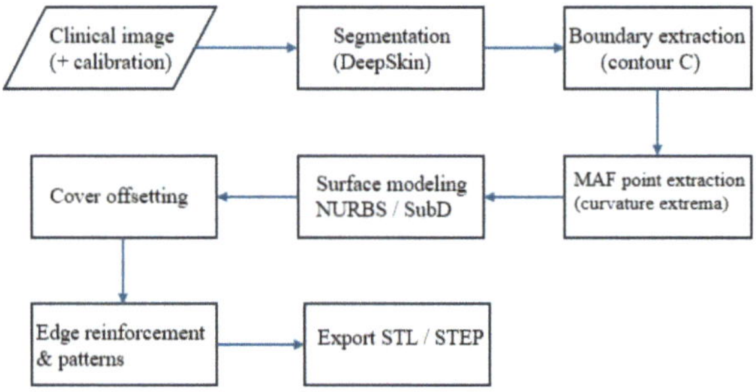

Fig. 5. Workflow for personalized cover generation from segmented wound surfaces. A curved anatomical surface is reconstructed and then converted into a thin, flexible shell by normal offsetting.

3 Results

3.1 Segmentation and MAF Extraction Results

The DeepSkin model achieved robust boundary segmentation, with average Dice coefficient of 0.93 ± 0.02 and mean boundary error of 0.4 mm, as supported by the contours shown in Fig. 1. The MAF reduction process condensed $\sim$ 1000 contour points into 15–25 control points, achieving $\approx 95\%$ data reduction. The MAF landmarks were consistently located at anatomically meaningful positions in multiple images, as illustrated in Figs. 2 and 3. In this study a total of 12 wound images were processed from 12 patients.

3.2 Surface Modeling Results

Both NURBS and SubD surfaces achieved sub-millimeter reconstruction accuracy. NURBS yielded slightly better RMS deviations for smooth geometries, while SubD performed better for lobed or asymmetric contours (Table 1).

Table 1. Surface deviation comparison between NURBS and SubD models.

Surface Type	RMS Deviation (mm)	Max Deviation (mm)
NURBS	0.41 ± 0.17	0.82 ± 0.26
SubD	0.46 ± 0.19	0.91 ± 0.33

Surfaces were generated in less than 5 s per case, ensuring near real-time performance. The qualitative comparison of surface smoothness and boundary adhesion is shown in Fig. 4.

3.3 Cover Generation Results

The offset produced thin-shell covers with uniform thickness (1.5–2.5 mm). For NURBS-based covers, the thickness deviation was 0.27 ± 0.09 mm, while SubD-based covers averaged 0.42 ± 0.13 mm due to the normal displacement of the vertex. Adaptive edges were correctly generated in high-curvature zones.

4 Discussions

The refined MAF workflow focuses on parametric surface modeling and cover generation, removing the lattice scaffold module to make the pipeline faster and easier to reproduce while maintaining sub-millimeter precision. These findings align with recent trends in CAD-based biomedical surface modeling and parametric implant design, which emphasize controllable, template-like representations for personalization [17], as well as advances in segmentation architectures, geometric deep learning on meshes and point sets, and CAD automation [18–26].

Advantages. The workflow achieves high accuracy (RMS deviation <0.5 mm between input and reconstructed surfaces), runs in less than 10 s per case, preserves topological stability across longitudinal updates through MAF anchors, and produces models that can be exported in STL/STEP format for 3D printing.

Limitations. Accuracy still depends on segmentation quality and image acquisition conditions; SubD offsetting can introduce small thickness variations due to vertex-normal displacement; and the limited dataset calls for further clinical validation on larger cohorts before routine deployment.

Future work will focus on automated optimization of ventilation patterns, integration with hybrid NURBS–SubD models, and expansion to craniofacial or orthopedic applications. In addition, the observed performance differences between NURBS and SubD suggest the potential for simple decision-support rules (e.g., curvature-or shape-complexity-based criteria) to automatically select the most appropriate surface representation for a given anatomy.

5 Conclusions

We present a refined and computationally efficient MAF-based workflow for anatomical surface reconstruction and personalized cover design. By integrating deep-learning segmentation, MAF-driven curvature analysis, and parametric modeling with NURBS and SubD surfaces, the approach achieves accurate and reproducible results suitable for additive manufacturing. The pipeline produces sub-millimeter precision, anatomical continuity, and manufacturable designs within seconds. The explicit description of NURBS parameterization, subdivision stopping criteria, and MAF thresholding further strengthens the reproducibility and potential for wider adoption of the proposed workflow.

Acknowledgements. This work was supported by the ERASMUS+ Partnerships for Cooperation and Exchange of Practices (KA220) project titled "Biomedical Innovations through Digital Transformation of Additive Technologies and Knowledge Exchange" — BIOMEDIX (Project No. 2024-1 LV01-KA220-HED-000255929). Financial support for publishing of this paper was ensured by the CNFIS-FDI-2025-F-0425 project titled "UTCN GLOBE – University without frontiers". Additional support was provided by the Science Fund of the Republic of Serbia (Project PRISMA, #7617), under the project titled "Multilevel approach to study chronic wounds based on clinical and biological assessment with development of novel personalized therapeutic approaches using in vitro and in vivo experimental models" — CHRONOWOUND.

References

1. Litjens G, Kooi T, Bejnordi BE et al (2017) A survey on deep learning in medical image analysis. Med Image Anal 42:60–88
2. Ronneberger O, Fischer P, Brox T (2015) U-net: convolutional networks for biomedical image segmentation. In: MICCAI, pp 234–241

3. Zhang H, Luo H, Hu Q (2022) Advanced wound dressings for chronic wounds: state of the art and future directions. Burns Trauma 10:tkac039
4. Ameer MA, Sharma S (2023) Wound dressings. In: StatPearls [internet]. StatPearls Publishing, Treasure Island, FL
5. Subagyo T, Ismail N, Ali M, Hassan M (2015) Geodesic path computation on trian- gular meshes for biomedical applications. J Comput Sci 11(5):792–802
6. Zheng Y, Yu J, Ma J et al (2018) Design and fabrication of porous scaffolds for tissue engineering using Voronoi diagram and 3D printing. J Mech Behav Biomed Mater 88:1–13
7. Attene M (2010) A lightweight approach to repairing digitized polygon meshes. Vis Comput 26:1393–1406
8. Klein A et al (2024) Comparative analysis of mesh vs. NURBS modeling in biomedical design. J Biomed Eng 51(2):205–219
9. Vitković N, Trajanović M, Stojkov S, Stanišić M (2013) Reverse engineering of hu- man bones by using method of anatomical features. FME Trans 41(4):310–316
10. Vitković N, Stanišić M, Trajanović M (2018) The method of anatomical features (MAF) for parametric modeling of human organs. CIRP Ann 67(1):173–176
11. Trajanović M, Vitković N, Manić M et al (2018) Automatic design of personalized lattice structures based on characteristic product features. CIRP Ann 67(1):181–184
12. Gibson I, Rosen DW, Stucker B (2015) Additive manufacturing technologies, 2nd edn. Springer, New York
13. ISO/ASTM 52900:2015 (2015) Additive manufacturing – general principles – terminology. ISO, Geneva
14. Duan X Accessed 2024: geomdl documentation. Available at: https://nurbs-python.readthedocs.io
15. Piegl L, Tiller W (1997) The NURBS book. Springer, Berlin
16. Catmull E, Clark J (1978) Recursively generated B-spline surfaces on arbitrary topological meshes. Comput Aided Des 10(6):350–355
17. Onal M et al (2023) Advances in CAD-based biomedical surface modeling. Comput Med Eng 47:101–115
18. Fang L et al (2025) Deep geometric processing of anatomical structures. Med Image Anal 89:102859
19. Fedorov A, Beichel R, Kalpathy-Cramer J et al (2012) 3D slicer as an image computing platform for the quantitative imaging network. Magn Reson Imaging 30(9):1323–1341
20. Kirillov, A.,(2023) et al: Segment anything arXiv:2304.02643
21. Cao H et al (2023) Swin-Unet: transformers for medical image segmentation. In: Proc. MICCAI
22. Qi CR et al (2023) Hierarchical deep learning on point sets in a metric space. Adv Geometric Deep Learning
23. Hanocka R et al (2023) MeshCNN: convolutional neural networks on meshes. ACM Trans Graph (TOG) 42(3)
24. Blender Foundation: Subdivision Surface Modeling Guide (2024) Blender Documentation
25. McNeel & Associates (2024) Rhino SubD technical documentation. Robert McNeel & Associates
26. Wang J et al (2024) Graph-based surface reconstruction for medical geometry. IEEE Access 12:55678–55690

A Proposal Model to Design an Emotional Assistance Robot to First Assistance at Health Area

Hector Cruz-Martinez, Leticia Neira-Tovar(✉), and Gabriel Monroy

Universidad Autonoma de Nuevo Leon, San Nicolas de Los Garza Nuevo Leon, Mexico
leticia.neiratv@uanl.edu.mx

Abstract. This paper presents the development of an emotionally intelligent robot system that integrates a language model (LLM) with computer vision–based emotion recognition to support basic healthcare interactions. The main objective was to design an empathetic conversational assistant capable of interpreting the user's emotional state and generating contextually appropriate verbal responses. The proposed system combines three main components: (1) a language-based voice assistant, (2) an emotion recognition module implemented with pretrained Python models, and (3) a multimodal interface running on a Raspberry Pi equipped with camera, microphone, and speakers. The implementation employs containerized environments and lightweight frameworks to ensure modularity, scalability, and local data processing. The integration of both components demonstrates the technical feasibility of creating low-cost, locally operated robots with emotional awareness. This work contributes to the field of affective computing by providing an accessible and adaptable framework for developing emotion-aware healthcare assistants.

Keywords: Assistance Robot · Lare Language Model · Emotion Recognition · LLM Agent · Healthcare · Artificial Intelligence

1 Introduction

1.1 An Introduction

In recent years, artificial intelligence has evolved to allow more natural and human interactions between people and machines. Large Language Models (LLMs) have driven the development of conversational assistants capable of understanding and generating language with a high level of contextual coherence. At the same time, computer vision has made it possible to identify human emotions through the analysis of facial expressions, generating useful applications in the educational, medical, and social assistance fields [1].

Initial Medical care not only requires technical skills but also empathy and effective communication with patients. In emergencies or first aid contexts, emotional support can reduce stress, stabilize the patient, and facilitate the work of medical personnel [2,

F. Górski et al. (Eds.): MANUFACTURING 2026, LNME, pp. 32–40, 2026.
https://doi.org/10.1007/978-3-032-23089-8_4

3]. In this context, artificial intelligence and emotional robotics offer new possibilities to provide psychological and communicative support during medical care [4, 5].

This Project seeks to unite these two areas, Large Language Models (LLMs) and computer vision, to create an empathetic emotional robot capable of recognizing human emotions and responding appropriately through text and voice [6, 7]. This work was carried out in the Virtual Reality Laboratory of Facultad de Ingenieria Mecanica y Electrica (UANL) and was structured in three phases:

1. Development of a lightweight language model for conversational interaction.
2. Implementation of the emotion recognition system in Python using pre-trained models.
3. Integration of both systems into a Raspberry Pi with interface and functional hardware.

1.2 Objective

The main objective is to demonstrate the technical and functional feasibility of an empathetic artificial intelligence system on accessible hardware, paving the wat for educational and social applications in affective robotics, as well as laying the foundation for future automated emotional assistance systems applicable in hospitals, rehabilitation centers, or first aid environments. Supported by the development and evaluation of an emotionally intelligent robotic assistant that integrates Large Language Models (LLMs) and computer vision to enable empathetic interaction and basic medical support [8]. Specifically, the study aims to demonstrate the technical and functional feasibility of combining a lightweight conversational model with an emotion recognition system capable of analyzing facial expressions and generating contextually appropriate verbal responses.

This work seeks to establish a modular and accessible architecture that operates entirely on local hardware, allowing for real-time interaction without reliance on external servers. By integrating language understanding and emotional perception into a single framework, the project contributes to the advancement of affective robotics and explores its potential applications in healthcare environments, such as patient assistance, rehabilitation support, and emergency response systems [9].

The system follows a decoupled architectural pattern Fig. 1 to ensure efficient emotional recognition. It begins with a Python Front End that captures and displays the user's emotions. This data is shared via RESTful API with the url /api/v1/promptMessage to a Spring Boot Back End, which serves as the orchestration layer. The core intelligence resides in the Ollama Agent Service (LLM), which receives the emotional context to generate suggestions. Finally, the response is sent back to the Python Front End to be transformed into audio. This structured flow ensures that the robot provides empathetic and context-aware responses, enhancing human-robot interaction.

2 Methodology

2.1 Phase 1: Implementation of the Large Language Model (LLM)

In the first phase, the artificial intelligence component responsible for robot communication was developed. Based on a language model (LLM). This module allows the robot to understand user questions and generate coherent and empathetic responses.

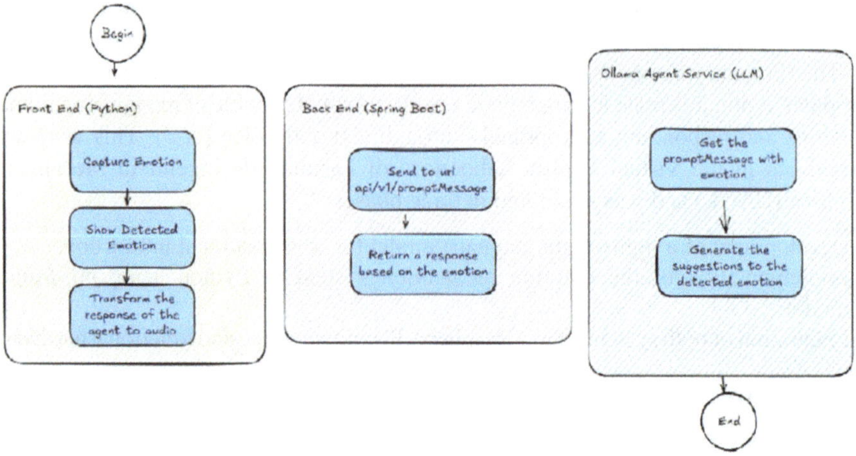

Fig. 1. Represents the flow chart of emotional robot recognition.

For this implementation, the Ollama environment was used, which allows lightweight language models to run locally, combining efficiency and low resource consumption. The model was deployed within a Docker environment, facilitating installation, portability, and compatibility with different systems.

In addition, a REST API was created using spring boot, enabling other components of the robot (such as the Raspberry Pi or the emotion recognition system) to communicate easily with the large language model. Interaction tests were carried out using Postman, verifying that the assistant's responses were coherent and contextual.

In this phase, the foundation of communication between the robot and the users was defined, establishing the basis for the conversational assistant that would later be integrated with the emotional vision system.

2.2 Phase 2: Emotion Recognition

The system was programmed in Python 3.10, using libraries such as TensorFlow/Keras for neural network modeling and OpenCV for real-time face detection through the camera [10–12]. The artificial intelligence model was trained from scratch using the FER-2013 dataset from Kaggle, which contains thousands of images labeled with seven emotions: anger, disgust, fear, happiness, sadness, surprise, and neutrality.

To improve accuracy, especially for emotions that are difficult to distinguish such as fear or anger, several advanced training techniques were implemented, including:

- Data Augmentation: creation of synthetic images with rotation, zoom, and translation to expand the dataset.
- Class Weights: compensation for underrepresented classes in the data.
- Batch Normalization: stabilization and acceleration of the training process.
- Adaptive Learning Rate (ReduceLROnPlateau): dynamic adjustment of the learning rate during optimization.

The training was carried out in Google Colab using GPU acceleration, and the resulting model was exported in keras format for later implementation on the Raspberry Pi. During execution, the system detects the user's face with OpenCV, processes the image, and displays the recognized emotion in real time through a simple visual interface.

The emotion recognition module sends the results to the language model (LLM), allowing the robot to adapt its tone and type of response according to the user's emotional state [13–17].

Future improvements include migrating to more modern face detectors such as MediaPipe, using more comprehensive datasets such as AffectNet or CK+, and optimizing performance with ONNX Runtime to reduce resource consumption [18].

The next figure (Fig. 2) represents the overall system, this architecture follows a modular and hierarchical organization that separates perceptual processing from cognitive reasoning, consistent with established design principles in computer vision and intelligent human–computer interaction, and enabling a clear methodological delineation between sensing, interpretation, and response generation.

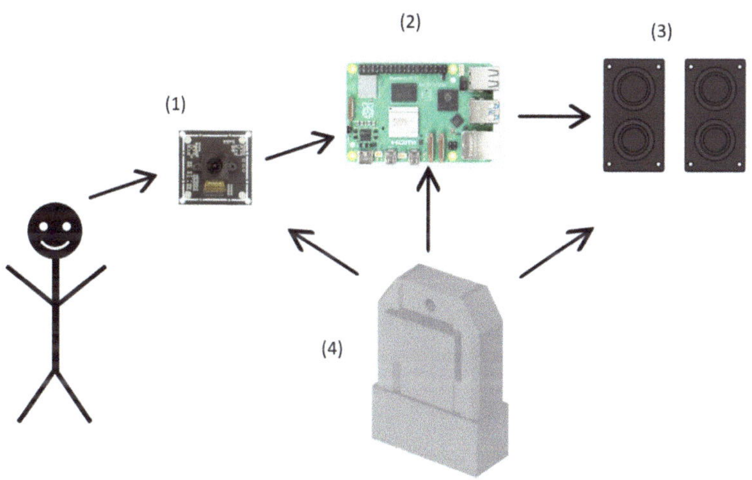

Fig. 2. Flow diagram of the components that involve emotion recognition.

2.3 Phase 3: Integration on Raspberry Pi

In the third phase, the complete integration between the physical hardware and the backend based on the Ollama API was carried out. The Raspberry Pi serves as the system's operating center, connecting the vision and language modules in a single functional environment.

The system installed on the Raspberry Pi sends requests to the Spring Boot–Ollama API service, which can run locally or on an external server within the same network. The interaction flow is structured as follows:

1. The camera captures the user's image and detects their emotions.

2. The Raspberry Pi sends the detected emotion to the REST API endpoint (/api/v1/generate).
3. The Ollama model processes the request and generates an empathetic recommendation or response based on the detected emotion.
4. The robot displays or reproduces the response through text or voice and stores the interaction in the database.

This modular design allowed asynchronous and secure communication between the Raspberry Pi and the artificial intelligence backend, taking advantage of containerization to ensure scalability, stability, and ease of maintenance.

The final integration that we showed in Fig. 3 combines emotional vision (Phase 2) with language (Phase 1), forming a complete emotional assistance system focused on supporting human interaction in healthcare environments.

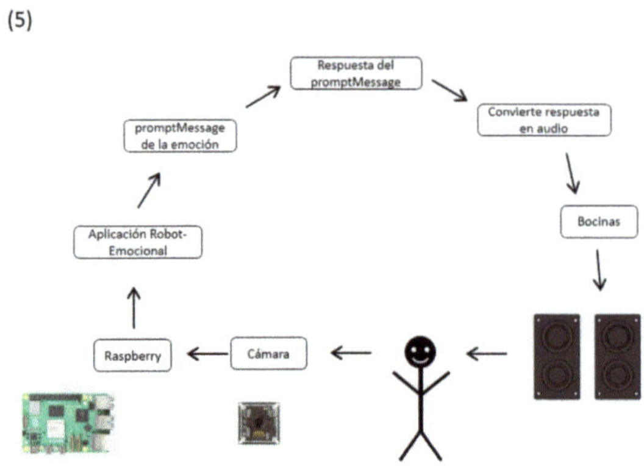

Fig. 3. The completed flow diagram of the integration of the emotional recognition robot is complete.

3 Results

The observed metrics validate the model's robust affective computing capabilities, achieving a 90% success rate in emotion recognition. This suggests that the underlying neural architecture effectively generalizes user emotional states. While process continuity was maintained in 83.3% of trials, the minor 16.7% latency rate indicates secondary hardware-software synchronization issues rather than a failure of the core AI logic (Fig. 4).

The integration on the Raspberry Pi made it possible to achieve a smooth execution of the complete system, with real-time emotion detection and coherent response generation by the conversational assistant. The language model operated efficiently through Docker, while emotion recognition achieved acceptable accuracy in classifying basic facial expressions.

During internal tests, it was verified that the system could react differently depending on the detected emotional state, showing basic empathetic behavior. In addition, the

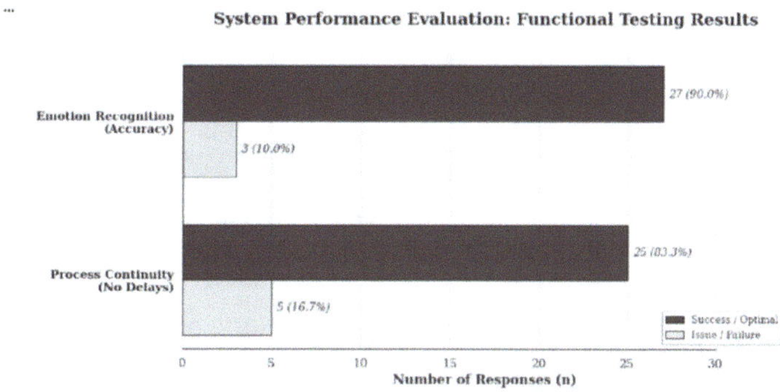

Fig. 4. Functional testing yielded a 90% emotion recognition accuracy and 83.3% process continuity.

voice interface showed good synchronization between recognition and speech synthesis, achieving natural interaction. This interaction between the visual and language modules was stable, demonstrating correct communication between the system components.

These results confirm the possibility of implementing empathetic artificial intelligence on low-cost platforms, with potential application in educational, therapeutic, and social assistance environments [19] (Figs. 5 and 6).

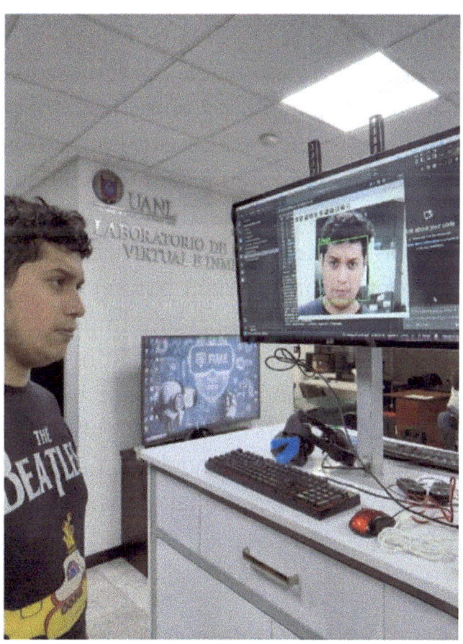

Fig. 5. The angry emotion recognition in production.

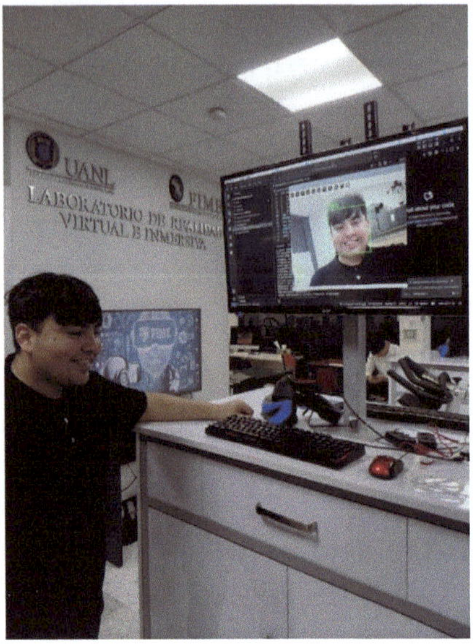

Fig. 6. The happy emotion recognition in production.

4 Conclusions

The development of this project made it possible to successfully integrate an emotional assistance system based on artificial intelligence, combining facial emotion recognition with a language model capable of generating empathetic responses [20]. The implementation on Raspberry Pi demonstrated that it is possible to run vision and language modules on low-cost hardware, maintain stable communication, and real-time response.

The use of Ollama, Docker, and Spring Boot facilitated the deployment of the language model, while TensorFlow and OpenCV enabled efficient visual processing for emotion detection. The connection between both systems consolidated a modular, flexible, and scalable architecture suitable for future improvements.

This work lays the foundation for the development of social robots with emotional capabilities, especially useful in health and first aid contexts, where empathy and communication can positively influence user well-being. As a future line of work, it is proposed to expand the emotional database, improve model training, and conduct user testing to evaluate the real impact of the robot in emotional assistance.

References

1. Agyei G, Ofori E, Asare A, Agyemang K (2025) Emotion-aware AI chatbots for mental health support in low-resource public health systems: a case study from Ghana. World J Public Health 10(3):17–29. https://doi.org/10.11648/j.wjph.20251003.17
2. Sociedad Española de Epidemiología (SEE). (2024). Libro de resúmenes: XLII Reunión Científica Anual de la Sociedad Española de Epidemiología y XVIII Congresso da Associação Portuguesa de Epidemiologia (AEP). https://www.reunionanualsee.org/documentos/Congreso%20SEE%202024.pdf

3. Sociedad Española de Médicos de Atención Primaria (SEMERGEN) (2020) Comunicado de la Sociedad Española de Médicos de Atención Primaria (SEMERGEN) en relación con la pandemia de COVID-19. Atención Primaria 52(4):282–283. https://doi.org/10.1016/j.aprim.2020.04.013
4. López-Gómez S, Pazo A (2023) The role of emotional intelligence and self-efficacy on the psychological well-being of university students. Psicodidáctica 28(2):163–171. https://doi.org/10.1016/j.psicod.2023.06.001
5. Muro C, Basterra RM, Cárdenas R, García TF, Giner EL (2012) Prevalencia de los trastornos de la personalidad en pacientes con trastornos de la conducta alimentaria. Revista de Psiquiatría y Salud Mental 5(1):13–20. https://doi.org/10.1016/j.rpsm.2011.11.001
6. Hernández JA, Calvo IL (2017) Detección de emociones en español a partir de texto y su aplicación en un agente conversacional. Revista Iberoamericana de Automática e Informática Industrial RIAI 14(4):427–436. https://polipapers.upv.es/index.php/RIAI/article/view/8277
7. Meenalochini P (2025) Emotion-aware conversational agents: affective computing using large language models and voice emotion recognition. J Art Intell Cyber Security (JAICS) 9(1) https://www.researchgate.net/publication/392522205_Emotion-Aware_Conversational_Agents_Affective_Computing_Using_Large_Language_Models_and_Voice_Emotion_Recognition
8. Lee JH, Kim JW, Lee SB (2025) The development of an emotional embodied conversational agent and the evaluation of the effect of response delay on user impression. Appl Sci 15(8):4256. https://doi.org/10.3390/app15084256
9. Gupta R, Cohen M, Sharma A (2025) Ethical considerations for empathetic AI in mental healthcare: a framework for development and deployment. Front Digital Health 7:1657031. https://doi.org/10.3389/fdgth.2025.1657031
10. Gupta R, Singh AK, Srivastava S, Dave R (2025) A comprehensive survey on multimodal emotion recognition from cognitive and physiological signals. Artif Intell Rev 58(5):131. https://doi.org/10.1007/s10462-025-11126-9
11. Gupta S, Sharma A, Verma RK, Singh PK (2025) Multi-modal emotion recognition using deep learning: a systematic review and future directions. Artif Intell Rev 58(7):198. https://doi.org/10.1007/s10462-025-11197-8
12. Wu Y, Liu S, Li J, Wang J, Zhang G (2025) A comprehensive review of multimodal emotion recognition: techniques, challenges, and future directions. Biomimetics 10(7):418. https://doi.org/10.3390/biomimetics10070418
13. Jia M, Sun Z (2024) A survey of multi-modal emotion recognition based on deep learning. Highlights Sci Eng Technol 119:533–540. https://www.researchgate.net/publication/387110436_A_Survey_of_Multi-modal_Emotion_Recognition_Based_on_Deep_Learning
14. Khan SH, Shah SAA, Bhatti MH, Anwar SM (2025) A survey on deep learning-based multimodal emotion recognition: modalities, fusion methods, and applications. IEEE Access 13:58498–58522. https://doi.org/10.1109/ACCESS.2025.3534197
15. Li Y, Zhang H, Wang Y, Liu J (2025) A multimodal emotion recognition framework based on feature fusion and transformer. In: 2025 International conference on artificial intelligence and computer applications (ICAICA). https://doi.org/10.1109/ICAICA.2025.10893614
16. Liu J, Zhang Y, Wang Y, Zhao G (2024) A novel multimodal emotion recognition method based on deep forest with hierarchical feature fusion. Expert Syst Appl 251:123261. https://doi.org/10.1016/j.eswa.2024.123261
17. Wang H, Wu Z, Li W, Pan J, Sun T (2024) A survey on multimodal emotion recognition: from features, models to applications. IET Collaborative Computational Project 6(1):e12116. https://doi.org/10.1049/ccs2.12116
18. Lee S, Kim SP, Thong DM, Seo M (2025) Empathetic conversational agents: utilizing neural and physiological signals for enhanced empathetic interactions. Int J Human–Computer Interaction. https://doi.org/10.1080/10447318.2025.2540500

19. Herath R (2025) Emotionally intelligent Chatbots in mental health: a review of psychological, ethical, and developmental impacts. Int J Comput Appl 187(29):49–56. https://www.researchgate.net/publication/394775017_Emotionally_Intelligent_Chatbots_in_Mental_Health_A_Review_of_Psychological_Ethical_and_Developmental_Impacts
20. Poria A, Chhaya G, Bafna R, Goel V (2024) A survey on empathetic conversational agents: from models to applications. Wiley Interdisciplinary Reviews: Data Mining and Knowledge Discovery 14(3):e1563. https://doi.org/10.1002/widm.1563

Intelligent and Automated Manufacturing Systems for Medical Applications

A Novel Method for Increasing the Accuracy of the WAAM Process Technology

Stefan Bodi(✉), Amina Vildanova, Zsolt-Levente Buna, Radu Comes, Călin Neamțu, Daniela Popescu, and Raul-Silviu Rozsos

Technical University of Cluj-Napoca, 103-105 Muncii Blvd., Cluj-Napoca 400641, Romania
stefan.bodi@muri.utcluj.ro

Abstract. Wire Arc Additive Manufacturing, a 3D printing technology that uses metal as base material, rose in popularity over the past few years due to the overall maturing of the 3D printing concept and the possibility of rapidly obtaining prototypes in an ever-growing competitive industrial environment. Yet, there are still a lot of shortcomings when employing this technology, that limit its applicability. This paper proposes a novel methodology that improves the accuracy of the WAAM process (employing an industrial robot) and the product's fidelity in relation to the 3D model, by scanning each printed layer and actively adjusting the printing / welding parameters (e.g. material feeding speed, robot speed, accuracy, acceleration, feedstock radius, material type, etc.), such that the prototype's shape will have a lower deviation in relation to the reference 3D model.

Keywords: Rapid prototyping · Additive manufacturing · WAAM · 3D printing · weld tracking system

1 Introduction

Wire Arc Additive Manufacturing (WAAM) is a rapid prototyping technology, that is based on depositing multiple metal layers through a consumable wire (as feedstock), melted down by an electric arc. The heated wire is transferred to the melt pool, where, after cooling, it solidifies and forms the designed part, layer by layer [1], as shown in Fig. 1.

WAAM technology offers several advantages: it's cost-effective since wire feedstock is considerably less expensive than powdered materials employed in other additive manufacturing processes; it enables high deposition rates, allowing for the rapid production of large-scale parts; it's readily available and flexible for printing workpieces with complex geometries; the waste resulting from this manufacturing process is relatively reduced, thus it's also environmentally friendly; finally, it allows the ability to repair or refurbish parts, that otherwise would be considered as scrap.

Beyond the technological advantages mentioned earlier, WAAM has become a focal point in digital manufacturing research because of its compatibility with Industry 4.0 principles. The process naturally generates large volumes of data related to thermal behavior, bead morphology, layer deposition accuracy, and material properties. When

F. Górski et al. (Eds.): MANUFACTURING 2026, LNME, pp. 43–54, 2026.
https://doi.org/10.1007/978-3-032-23089-8_5

this information is integrated with modern sensing technologies, WAAM can function as a fully cyber-physical process where each manufacturing step is monitored, validated, and corrected in real time. This paradigm shift from traditional open-loop welding to intelligent closed-loop additive manufacturing creates new opportunities for quality assurance and automation.

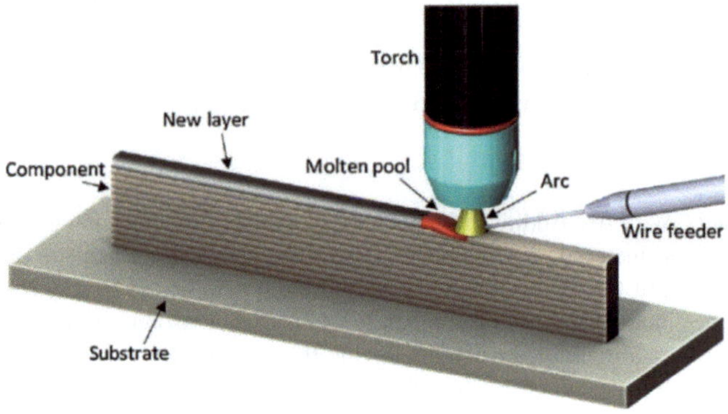

Fig. 1. WAAM printing process [2]

Furthermore, as industries transition toward more sustainable production models, WAAM offers a compelling path due to its minimal material waste and potential for part repair. The ability to reconstruct damaged components, such as turbine blades or structural brackets, reduces the environmental burden associated with producing replacements. These trends reinforce the need for more accurate deposition strategies, since higher repeatability and dimensional control directly influence how easily WAAM can be adopted for safety-critical or high-value components.

In a WAAM system, mostly industrial robots are used, due to their precise control, flexibility, scalability, endurance (in a manufacturing environment) and ability to enhance safety. In addition, robots allow a more accurate deposition (compared to other available WAAM solutions) [3], can work on various part geometries, and can be integrated seamlessly into existing production lines. Robots improve productivity, ensure dimensional accuracy, and provide efficient scalability in manufacturing [4].

However, one of the main drawbacks of WAAM technology is the inferior surface quality of the printed parts. The deposition process can result in a rough surface finish, which may require additional (multiple) finishing steps to achieve the desired surface quality [5]. An example of a WAAM printed part before and after post-processing is illustrated in Fig. 2.

Various methods can be adopted to improve the surface quality in WAAM, such as: material selection – choosing smoother starting materials for the wire; process optimization – adjusting printing welding parameters (such as, material feeding rate, robot speed, accuracy, acceleration, feedstock radius, etc.) [7]; tool path optimization – optimizing the robot's tool center point (TCP) reduces surface roughness; continuous monitoring – layer-by-layer monitoring identifies defects for immediate correction, feedstock refining, heat management; etc.

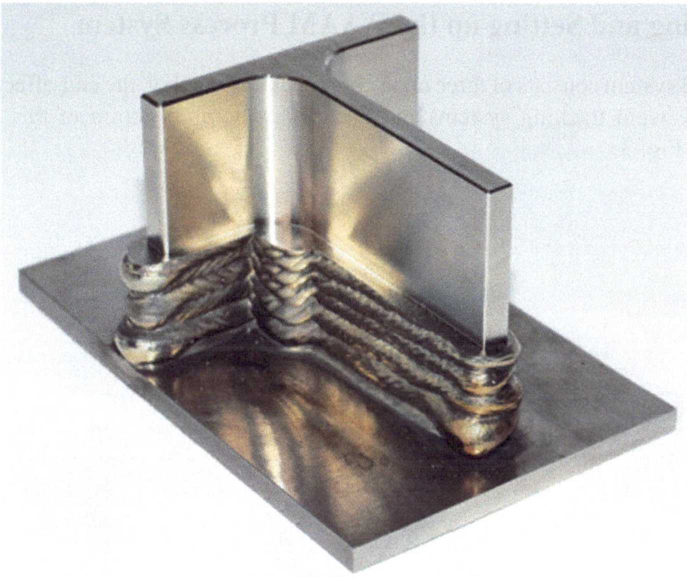

Fig. 2. WAAM printed part before (bottom) and after (top) post-processing [6]

The authors propose a system that focuses on the later method, namely, the layer-by-layer monitoring is completed by employing a 3D scanner, attached to the end-effector, such that it can track how the printing /welding process is performing. By doing so, if larger deviations are identified, printing parameters are adjusted, such that the printed layer has a higher degree of fidelity with the 3D model's surface.

The reasons behind this approach are summed up as follows:

- Ensuring surface quality: by scanning the surface after each layer deposition, any defects, deviations, or irregularities can be detected early in the process; this allows for taking immediate corrective measures and ensuring a better surface quality;
- Process control: the scanning of each layer generates high volumes of data that can be compared to the CAD data, and if the case, adjustments can be made as the printing process is ongoing, in real-time, to obtain a more accurate layer deposition;
- Error detection and correction: scanning helps identify any errors or issues that may occur during the printing process; by detecting these problems early on, appropriate actions can be taken to rectify them, minimizing the chances of propagating errors throughout subsequent layers;
- Optimization and parameter tuning: after the printing process for the first workpiece is completed, the scanning data of each layer can be analyzed for highly tuning the printing / welding parameters, such that the following workpieces that are printed have a higher dimensional accuracy and a better surface fidelity;
- Process documentation and traceability: digital records of the manufacturing process' performance are obtained in the form of scanning data, which enables traceability and facilitates the validation of the manufacturing process.

2 Devising and Setting up the WAAM Process System

The devised system consists of three main components: the robot, the end-effector (welding torch & weld tracking system) and the CPU. The architecture of this system is depicted in Fig. 3.

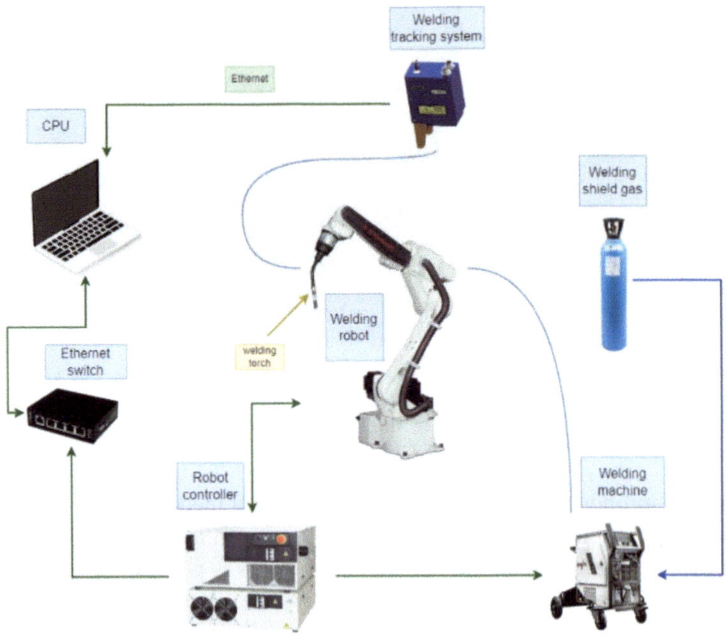

Fig. 3. WAAM printing system's architecture

2.1 The Robot

The Kawasaki BA006N welding robot was deemed appropriate for this application considering its ruggedness, accuracy, versatility, advanced control system, user-friendly interface, and reliable support. The robot is paired with an EWM Titan XQ welding power source and its controller is equipped with Ethernet, USB, and RS-232C ports. Its setup can be seen in Fig. 4.

The choice of robot architecture plays a defining role in the stability of WAAM deposition. Industrial welding robots such as the Kawasaki BA006N offer smooth trajectory execution and consistent velocity control, both of which are critical for ensuring uniform bead morphology. Even small fluctuations in TCP speed can lead to underfill, overfill, or asymmetrical bead shapes. By selecting a robot equipped with advanced motion control algorithms and high repeatability, the deposition process becomes more predictable and easier to adjust dynamically. Additionally, the robot's ability to execute non-linear toolpaths makes it suitable for components with varying curvature or multi-directional printing strategies, which are becoming increasingly common in WAAM applications.

Another important aspect is the integration capability between the robot controller and external sensing systems. The architecture used in this work allows synchronized data acquisition at the moment of layer scanning, enabling accurate pairing between robot pose information and sensor output. This synchronization is essential for reconstructing the real geometry of each layer without temporal displacement errors between the robot's movement and the sensor's sampling behavior.

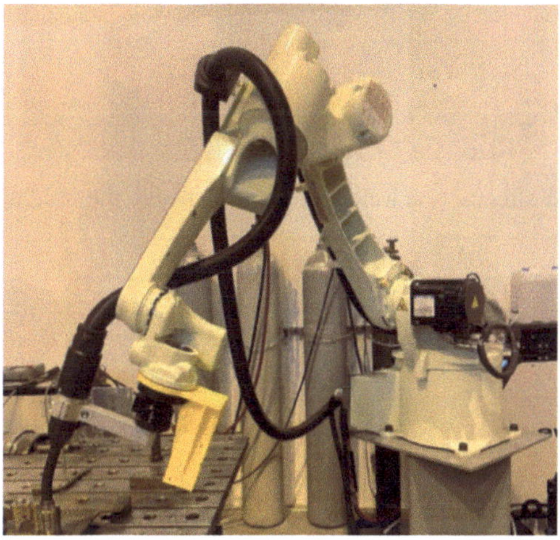

Fig. 4. Kawasaki BA006N paired with an EWM Titan XQ welding power source

2.2 The End-Effector

As seem in Fig. 4, to the Kawasaki BA006N is attached an end-effector that is comprised of two parts linked together with a fastener: the welding torch and the weld tracking system (Fig. 5). The welding torch performs the addition of material, while the weld tracking system enables the evaluation of the profile, resulting from the weld.

2.3 The CPU

The CPU acts as a client that collects data packets: the first one is comprised of an array of X and Z coordinates (data from the weld tracking system), while the second one contains the Y coordinates (obtained from the robot's movement, while scanning each layer). Combining the two arrays, results in a point cloud, corresponding to each of the printing layers (Fig. 6).

The processing pipeline implemented at the CPU level is pivotal for transforming raw sensor data into a meaningful geometric description. Beyond simple data merging, pre-processing steps such as noise removal, smoothing, and outlier detection help ensure that the resulting point cloud accurately represents the deposited bead. Variations in reflectivity, molten metal brightness, or local overheating can lead to measurement

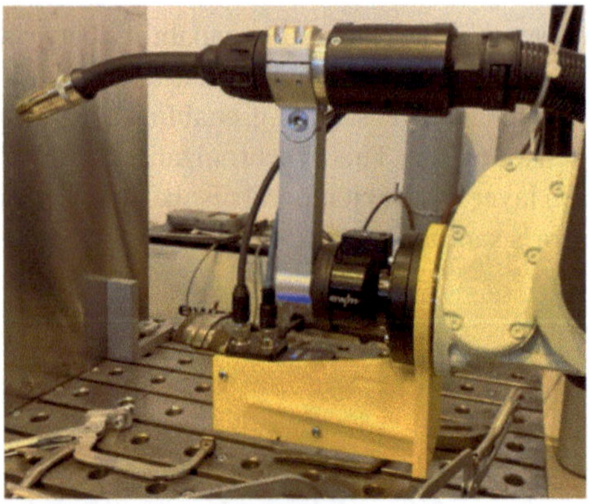

Fig. 5. The end-effector (the welding torch attached to the weld tracking system)

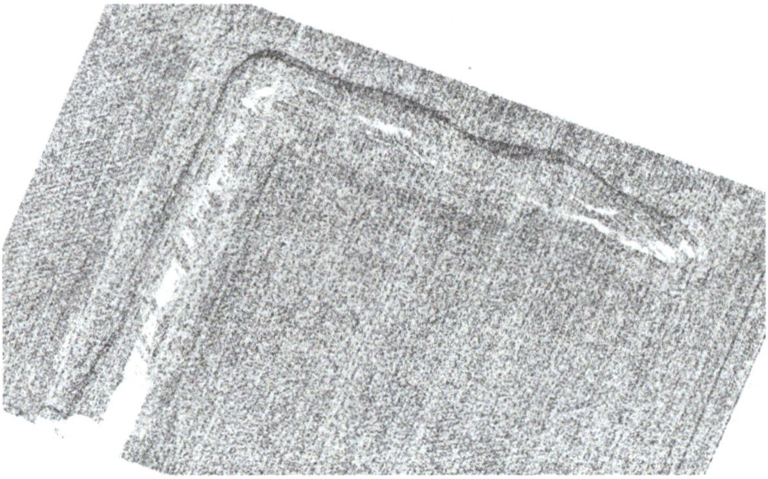

Fig. 6. Example of point cloud for the first printed layer

artefacts, so robust filtering strategies are required to extract usable information from each scan. Once processed, the point cloud serves as a detailed digital fingerprint of that specific layer.

A key advantage of this digital reconstruction is the ability to perform automatic cross-section evaluation. By comparing the scanned bead geometry to the theoretical model, the system can detect whether the printed layer is too high, too wide, or insufficiently filled. This automated geometric characterization forms the basis for adaptive parameter correction in the following deposition step and demonstrates the potential of combining sensor-guided metrology with WAAM.

3 Experimental Results

In order to highlight the capabilities of the devised system, a simpler workpiece was modeled for the WAAM process, as shown in Fig. 7. Its dimensions are 100 mm by 100 mm with a 90° angle and 50 mm in height.

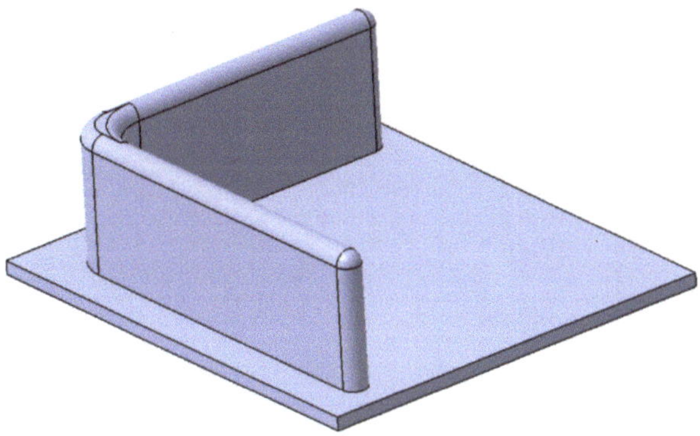

Fig. 7. 3D model of the designed workpiece

The 3D printing process was started with the following parameters:

- Wire: austenitic stainless steel of grade AISI 310;
- Welding type: MIG (mechanized welding with a melting electrode in an inert gas - Argon - environment);
- Wire feed speed: 4.5 m/min;
- Speed of surfacing (robot movements): 90 cm/min;
- Current: 139A;
- Voltage: 18.0 V (Fig. 8)

After the first layer was completed and the layer cooled down the scanning process was deployed (Fig. 9) to check the results and perform a deviation analysis.

The scanning step, performed after each cooling cycle, provides crucial insight into how thermal gradients influence bead deformation. Since WAAM inherently involves cyclic heating and cooling, each newly deposited layer imposes additional thermal stress on the previous ones. This effect may lead to local distortions, warping, or bead collapse if not properly monitored. The scanning process captures these thermal-induced geometric changes, allowing the system to identify whether the deviation originates from deposition parameters or from heat accumulation within the structure.

Another advantage of layer scanning lies in its capacity to detect anomalies that are not visible to the naked eye. Minor shifts in bead symmetry, local undercuts, or asymmetrical spreading of molten metal can serve as early indicators of future defects. Detecting these issues layer-by-layer prevents the amplification of errors in higher layers and significantly enhances the overall print stability.

In the point clouds extra data was obtained such as points of the substrate on which the metal was surfaced. This information was further filtered (through 3 steps) and only

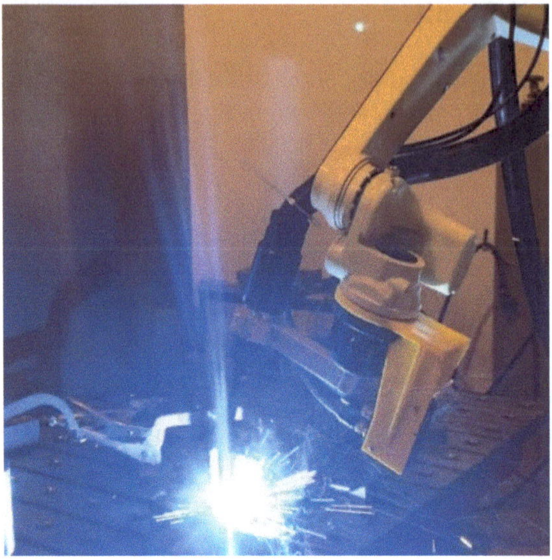

Fig. 8. WAAM process

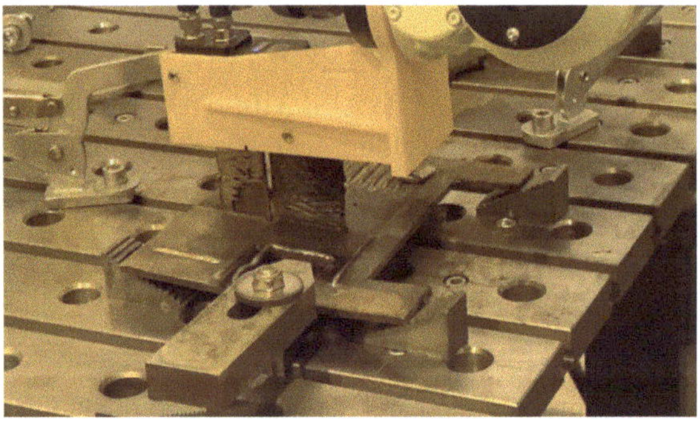

Fig. 9. Scanning of the first layer

the polygonal models in the immediate vicinity of the layers were considered (as shown in Fig. 10).

The resulting mesh (final scan data) was subsequently analyzed by inserting side and top section planes, and by extracting the profiles of the layer transversely and lengthwise, as shown in Figs. 11 and 12

The use of section planes for mesh analysis creates a systematic framework for evaluating layer consistency. By slicing the point cloud into transversal and longitudinal sections, the system can compare the obtained layer profiles against the theoretical CAD boundaries with high precision. This comparison enables the calculation of deviation maps, highlighting local overbuilt or underbuilt regions. Such detailed geometric feedback is essential for refining the WAAM process, especially when printing components with demanding tolerance requirements.

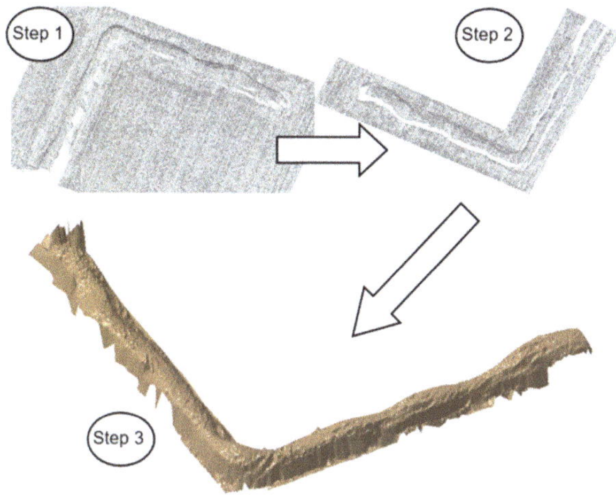

Fig. 10. Filtering scanned data

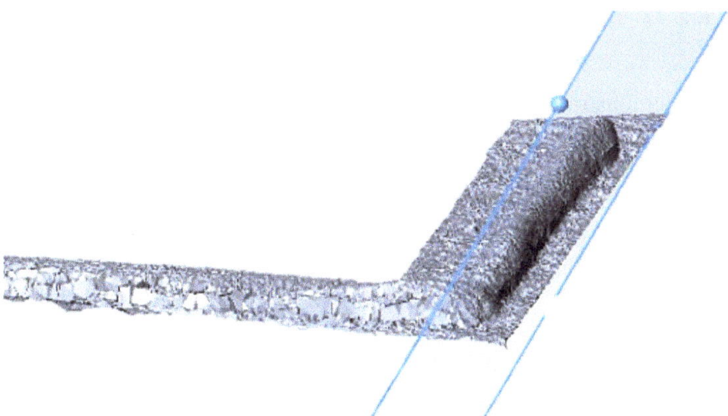

Fig. 11. Creating section planes through the obtained mesh

Moreover, the multi-directional sectioning method helps capture the asymmetric nature of bead formation, which often varies based on torch angle, travel speed, and heat input distribution. Traditional WAAM evaluation methods rely primarily on visual inspection or isolated cross-section cuts, whereas the method described here offers full-field information without destroying the workpiece. This allows for comprehensive monitoring while maintaining the continuity of the print.

The extracted profiles were compared with profiles from the theoretical 3D model and sections that had a larger deviation were isolated. For the identified "problem-sections" the WAAM process parameters were adjusted accordingly, to compensate for the errors on each of the 10 layers, depending on the error in question.

This approach was repeated 10 times, one time for each layer, thus an equal number of point clouds were also obtained / analyzed.

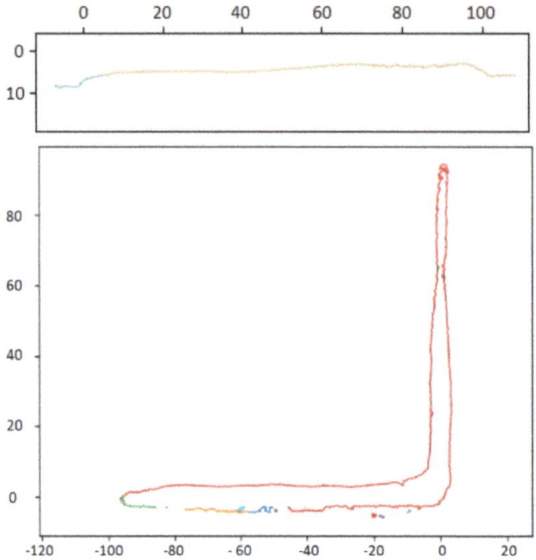

Fig. 12. Extracting profiles by intersecting the mesh and section planes

Finally, to demonstrate the capabilities of this methodology, another part was printed / welded, however in this case the parameters were not modified in any way. Fig. 13 and 14 illustrate the differences between the two approaches, and it can be clearly seen that the workpiece printed by employing the methodology proposed by the authors is of higher surface fidelity with the 3D model.

It should be noted, that even if the workpiece obtained by employing the proposed methodology still requires some final finishing operations, yet they are minor, thus the costs associated with them are reduced, they take up less time and the overall prototyping process is shortened considerably.

The comparative analysis between the adaptively controlled workpiece and the one produced with unmodified parameters illustrates the direct impact of closed-loop monitoring on surface fidelity. The deviations observed in the unmodified print demonstrate how cumulative errors propagate when the deposition process is not continuously corrected. Minor bead height variations on the initial layers grow into pronounced distortions as the structure increases in height. These deviations are particularly visible along the edges and corners, where thermal accumulation tends to be more significant.

In contrast, the adaptively corrected workpiece shows much more stable bead stacking and uniformity. Even though small imperfections remain, their magnitude is significantly reduced, enabling a shorter and more efficient post-processing stage. This improvement highlights the potential of integrating sensor feedback into existing WAAM systems and represents an important step toward autonomous additive welding processes capable of meeting industrial accuracy requirements.

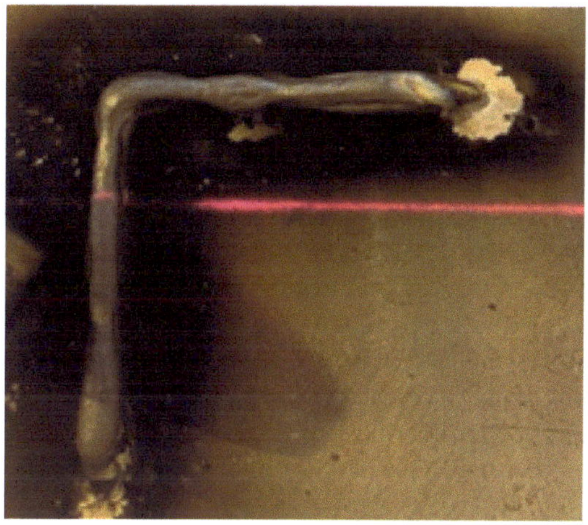

Fig. 13. Workpiece obtained by employing the proposed methodology

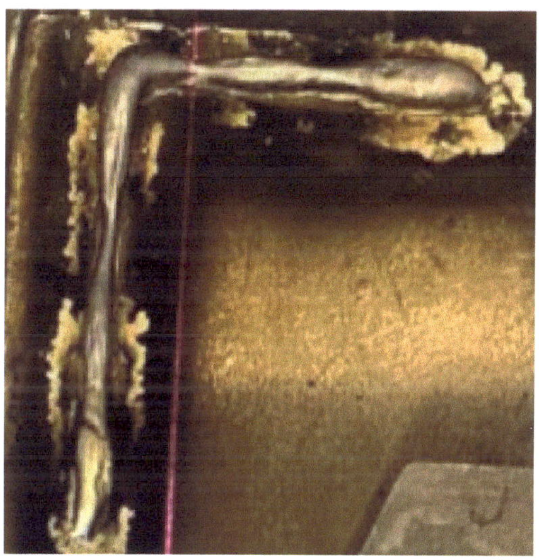

Fig. 14. Workpiece obtained with unmodified WAAM process parameters

4 Conclusions

In this paper, a novel method was proposed for increasing the accuracy and fidelity of workpieces printed / welded using the WAAM process. The architecture of the proposed system permitted the extension of such a technology with scanning techniques, thus enabling the verification of each layer. By doing so, proper corrective actions could be taken in due time, early on in the process, by adjusting the parameters, such that the final workpiece would require fewer finishing operations, to save time and costs related to the prototyping process.

The results obtained confirm that integrating 3D scanning into the WAAM workflow can substantially reduce geometric deviations by enabling real-time or near-real-time parameter adjustments. The methodology demonstrates how sensor-augmented additive manufacturing can evolve from a passive deposition system into an active, self-correcting platform. While the current system focuses on layer geometry, future developments may include thermal field monitoring, melt pool shape analysis, or machine-learning-based prediction models that anticipate deviations before they occur.

Additionally, the experimental findings suggest that the approach is scalable and may be adapted to a wide range of materials and component sizes. By reducing the need for extensive post-processing and increasing shape fidelity, the proposed methodology contributes to lowering manufacturing costs and improving production throughput. Continued research in this direction may pave the way for fully autonomous WAAM pipelines capable of producing near-net-shape parts with minimal human intervention.

References

1. Shahir MY, Cutler S, Nong G (2019) Review: the impact of metal additive manufacturing on the aerospace industry. Metals 9(12):art. no. 1286
2. Rodrigues TA, Duarte V, Miranda RM, Santos TG, Oliveira JP (2019) Current status and perspectives on wire and arc additive manufacturing (WAAM). Materials 12(7):art. no. 1121
3. Wang X, Fang P, Teng B, Xu K, Sun H, Wang X (2020) Design of WAAM system based on industrial robot. In: Chen S, Zhang Y, Feng Z (eds) Transactions on intelligent welding manufacturing, vol 4, No. 2. Springer, Heidelberg, pp 91–106
4. Arana M, Ukar E, Rodriguez I, Iturrioz A, Alvarez P (2021) Strategies to reduce porosity in Al-Mg WAAM parts and their impact on mechanical properties. Metals 11(3):art. no. 524
5. Cunningham CR, Flynn JM, Shokrani A, Dhokia V, Newman ST (2018) Invited review article: strategies and processes for high quality wire arc additive manufacturing. Addit Manuf 22:672–686
6. Gross Publications, Inc (2020) Wire Arc additive manufacturing. Available online at: https://mfgnewsweb.com/archives/4/57088/Advanced-Mfg-Solutions-aug20/Wire-Arc-Additive-Manufacturing.aspx. Last accessed 13 Nov 2025
7. Nguyen VT et al (2023) AAM technique: process parameters affecting the mechanical properties and microstructures of low-carbon steel. Metals 13(5):art. no. 873

Simulation Analysis of a Robotic Workplace for Additive Manufacturing of Dental Implants

Maryna Yeromina(✉), Jozef Török, Samuel Mikuláško, and Darina Dupláková

Faculty of Manufacturing Technologies with a Seat in Presov, Technical University of Košice, Prešov 080 01, Slovakia
maryna.yeromina@tuke.sk

Abstract. This article presents an integrated approach to the design and evaluation of an automated workplace to produce dental implants, combining the implementation of industrial robots, the safety requirements of ISO 10218-1 and modern additive manufacturing technologies. The article focuses on the implementation of an industrial robot in accordance with the standard, which sets out key principles for the safe operation of robotic systems in automated production environments. The work also includes an overview of advanced 3D printing technologies used in dentistry, in particular SLS and SLM methods, which enable the production of precise and individually tailored implants with high material efficiency. A virtual model of the workplace was created in Tecnomatix Plant Simulation software, consisting of a 3D metal printer, a cleaning station, finishing technology and an industrial robot for handling parts and connecting individual operations. The simulation model is used to analyse the dynamic behaviour of the system, its capacity utilisation and operational performance. The simulation outputs include Resource Statistics, Occupancy and Active Work Share pie charts, which enabled detailed identification of inactivity, potential bottlenecks and overall resource utilisation. The results confirm the suitability and effectiveness of linking industrial robotics with additive manufacturing technologies in the dental implant manufacturing process. The findings also highlight the importance of simulation tools in verifying workplace design before its actual implementation.

Keywords: Robotic Workplace · Additive Manufacturing · Dental Implants · Simulation · Analysis

1 Introduction

In today's industry, there has been a significant increase in the use of automation and robotic technologies, which are gradually taking over tasks traditionally performed by humans. Industrial robots are increasingly being deployed for operations requiring high repeatability, precision or physical exertion.

F. Górski et al. (Eds.): MANUFACTURING 2026, LNME, pp. 55–69, 2026.
https://doi.org/10.1007/978-3-032-23089-8_6

1.1 Implementation of Industrial Robots in Machining Processes

Modern robotic systems achieve a level of movement flexibility comparable to that of humans and enable the performance of more complex tasks. Research shows [1] that the introduction of robotisation can lead to an increase in productivity of approximately 30%, a reduction in production costs of up to 50% and the achievement of more than 85% capacity utilisation. However, the implementation of robotic solutions is associated with high investment costs and is therefore only economically viable under certain conditions – particularly in large-scale production, highly repetitive and precise activities, or in environments that pose a risk to human workers. Such conditions are typical, for example, in the automotive industry, which is also the largest user of industrial robots [2]. Modern production systems are characterised by a high degree of complexity, which makes their analysis significantly more difficult. A wide range of methodologies are therefore used to solve such tasks, including mathematical modelling, combinatorial optimisation, Petri nets and scenario analysis [3]. Among these, computer simulation methods are the most widely used, especially discrete event simulation (DES), which is considered the most versatile and frequently used approach. There are a number of manufacturing-oriented DES software packages on the market, such as ARENA, Enterprise Dynamics, FlexSim, Plant Simulation, SIMIO, and Witness [4]. The key advantage of DES is the ability to perform a large number of experiments in a short time, many of which would not be possible on a real production system due to operational constraints or the high cost of industrial equipment. The simulation model provides important insights that can subsequently contribute to improving the actual system [3]. A disadvantage of DES is the presence of random variables, which can sometimes make it difficult to distinguish whether the results are caused by system dynamics or randomness [3]. The creation of complex production systems requires the harmonisation of several areas – production strategies, system architecture, capacity planning, control techniques, performance evaluation methods, scenario analysis and risk assessment [5]. The design process begins with conceptual modelling, which involves defining the problem and identifying system constraints. At this stage, it is necessary to specify what will be modelled and how [6]. To support conceptual design, it is often recommended to use graphical diagram methods [4], such as object flow diagrams (OFD) [6]. Classic automated manufacturing systems are primarily designed for mass production, where component uncertainty plays a significant role. However, in the early stages of system design, it is often very difficult to reliably estimate its future reliability [7]. The transition to flexible and intelligent robotic systems is considered a key step towards Industry 4.0 [5]. In some applications, robots and humans can work together, but this requires a very high level of safety. Collaborative robots only meet these requirements when operating at low speeds [8]; therefore, industrial robots are usually placed in fenced cells, which allow high performance to be achieved while being completely separated from human operators. The main steps of the proposed methodology are shown in Fig. 1. They include analysis of the real problem, conceptual design and creation of a simulation model, performing simulation experiments to find a solution, and then implementing the solution in practice.

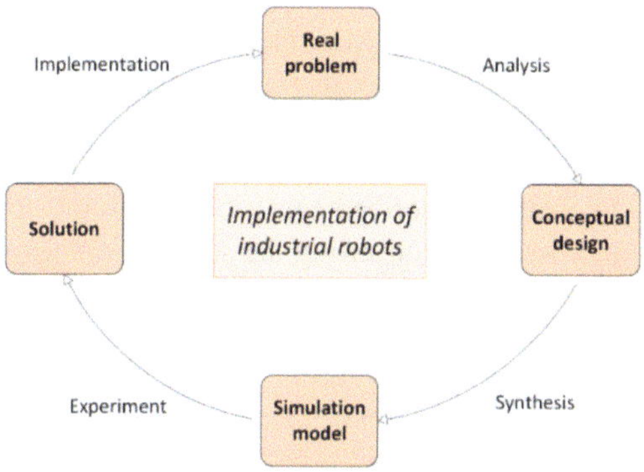

Fig. 1. Methodology for implementing an industrial robot.

1.2 Standards ISO 10218-1

The STN EN ISO 10218-1 standard deals with safety requirements for the use of industrial robots in automated production. Its main objective is to define procedures and rules that will ensure the protection of workers and reduce the risk of accidents associated with the operation of robotic systems. The standard specifies the requirements for the construction, design and placement of industrial robots in specific operating conditions. It focuses primarily on the safety of people who may come into contact with the robot during maintenance, inspection or servicing of automated production lines. Key areas addressed by the standard include protective measures for robotic equipment, procedures for ensuring safe operation, and recommendations for the planning and installation of robotic systems. Thanks to its comprehensive safety framework, the STN EN ISO 10218-1 standard contributes to the safe and effective integration of industrial robots into production processes, while protecting the health and safety of workers operating in the vicinity of automated technologies [9].

1.3 3D Technologies in the Manufacture of Dental Implants

Additive manufacturing (AM) has brought new possibilities to dentistry, as 3D printing technologies have gradually enabled more accurate, faster and more cost-effective treatments [10]. A key element of AM is computer-aided design (CAD), which enables the creation of digital models for 3D printing with minimal material waste. This approach contrasts with traditional subtractive manufacturing methods. Additive manufacturing also allows for the processing of various types of materials, such as metals, ceramics and thermoplastic resins [10].

The concept of hybrid materials and hybrid manufacturing processes, which was analysed in detail by Silvo et al. [11], is known from several technical fields, such as electronics and aerospace. In dentistry, these approaches are used to eliminate problems associated with tooth loss and to improve the quality, efficiency and economy of dental prostheses. Hybrid techniques offer a high degree of freedom in designing individual geometries and combining different materials. The literature discusses new processes using a combination of several AM technologies, in particular selective laser melting

(SLM) (Fig. 2), selective laser sintering (SLS) (see Fig. 2) [12]. The spontaneous formation of fractal-type structures at the mesoscale is also mentioned as a promising direction of research in implant design [13]. The advantage of combining multiple AM methods is the achievement of high mechanical strength and an optimal weight-to-volume ratio of the final product. The method described consisted of several steps: (1) scanning the area of the jaw with tooth loss, (2) converting the scans into uneven rational B-splines for further processing in 3D CAD software, followed by the design of a customised implant using 3D techniques and topological optimisation. The core of the implant, made of metal or ceramic material, provides the necessary mechanical strength, while the polymer surface gives it suitable biomechanical properties.

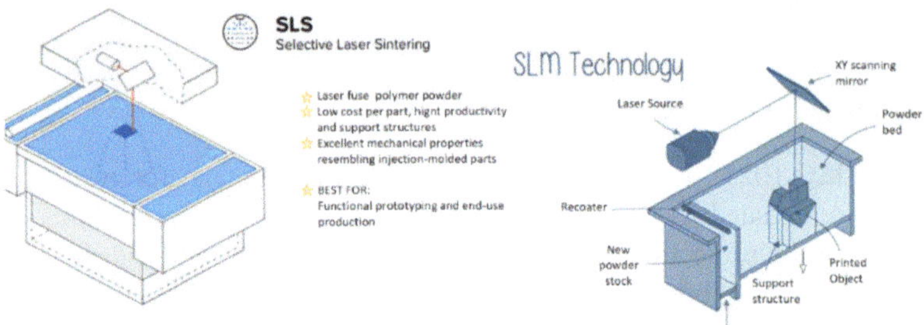

Fig. 2. Additive technologies used in dental implant production.

Selective Laser Sintering (SLS) is an additive manufacturing technology in which a laser sinteres powdered material (most often polymers) into a solid layer without completely melting the particles. Selective Laser Melting (SLM) is a similar process, but in this case the laser completely melts the metal powder, creating a highly homogeneous and solid metal component with properties comparable to cast or machined parts.

R. Ramakrishnaiah et al. [14], Patil et al. [15] and Kasambe et al. [16] attempted to produce dental implants from Ti-6Al-4 V using electron beam melting (EBM), which is an additive manufacturing method. The EBM method is used because it is suitable for the production of titanium alloys, which are generally difficult to work with because they are highly reactive at higher temperatures. EBM uses Ti-6Al-4 V powder in a vacuum, preventing reaction between the powder and air during production. The implant was evaluated based on parameters such as surface microstructure, topography, chemical composition, wettability, and internal microstructure. The model produced in the experiment shows an irregular side surface and a smoother surface of the structure. The rough surface allows for bone bonding, which can be beneficial, but also has the disadvantage of trapping food particles and other complications. Better wettability was found, which improved adhesion to implant surfaces. The model provided satisfactory results based on all of the above parameters and can be considered a good choice for the manufacture of custom dental implants [15].

2 Theoretical Background

The field of 3D printing of dental implants is dominated by literature focusing on materials, surface treatments and biological response. Alqutaibi et al. conducted an extensive review study of advanced additive technologies in implant dentistry, comparing different 3D printing technologies (SLM, EBM, DLP, etc.), printed materials and their mechanical and osseointegration properties. The authors point out that 3D-printed titanium implants can achieve mechanical properties comparable to conventionally machined implants, but they draw attention to the critical role of post-processing (heat treatment, polishing, surface modification) and the lack of standardised testing protocols [17]. Pradíes et al. conducted a scoping review of current applications of 3D printing in implantology, systematically mapping the use of 3D printing in the manufacture of implants, surgical templates and prosthetic superstructures. They conclude that 3D printing is already routinely used in the manufacture of templates and individual superstructures, while for implants themselves, clinical evidence is still fragmented and based mainly on small case studies or short-term follow-ups. The main weakness of the work is the high heterogeneity of the studies included – different technologies, materials, protocols and success metrics – which makes quantitative comparison and the creation of clear clinical recommendations difficult [18]. An important addition is the broader overview by Chen and Wei, who analyse the use of 3D printing in dentistry as a whole, including dental implants, prosthetics, orthodontics and tissue engineering. The authors emphasise the potential of personalised root-shaped implants and patient-specific designs, but also point out regulatory barriers, variable print quality between devices and insufficient integration of additive manufacturing into standardised digital workflows. It is important to note that this synthesis also lacks a description of fully automated, robotised production lines for implants, focusing instead on individual technological steps rather than a comprehensive robotic workplace [19]. When looking for analogies to robotic production workplaces, it is therefore necessary to turn to general industrial literature. Montini et al. present a case study of a collaborative robotic cell in an assembly process, where the main goal is not only to increase productivity but also to improve ergonomics and worker well-being. The work shows that a properly designed HRC (human-robot collaboration) can shorten cycle times and reduce the physical strain on operators, but implementation requires detailed risk analysis, repeated layout tuning and staff training. The limitation of the study is its focus on one small company and a specific product, which limits the direct generalisation of the results to other types of production, including medical devices [20]. At the level of synthesising reviews, Wang et al. address the issue of collaborative robots, summarising the state of knowledge in the field of surface and finishing operations in manufacturing. The authors emphasise that cobots enable flexible automation of small and medium series, but point out the limited number of systematic experimental studies, often only with technological metrics (cycle time, surface roughness), lacking a comprehensive assessment of economics, ergonomics and long-term reliability. From the perspective of this work, it is important that the review clearly shows the transferability of robotic cell design principles (layout, workplace sharing, safety zones, task planning) to highly regulated industries such as medical device manufacturing [21]. Barosz et al. analyse the efficiency of a machining line where parts are handled either by human operators or industrial robots. Based on discrete simulation in FlexSim and OEE/OFE indicators, they compare different line staffing options and show that the use of robots can significantly increase productivity and flow stability, while also pointing out the sensitivity of the system to robot failures and the need to consider reliability at the design stage. The study is strong in its detailed modelling of a real line in the automotive industry, but its conclusions are tied to a specific type of process and are not directly verified by long-term operational data [22]. Makulavičius focuses on industrial robots in the field of machining and provides an overview of the most common robotic operations (milling, drilling, grinding, polishing) with an emphasis on their limitations and possibilities for improvement. He emphasises that the key challenge is the low rigidity of the robotic structure and the associated accuracy; therefore, much of the research focuses on optimising the robot's position, tool trajectory and sensor integration with advanced control algorithms or machine learning. However, the author notes that many of the proposed solutions remain in the laboratory phase and that there is a lack of systematic industrial case studies of fully integrated robotic machining cells [23]. Karabegović et al. focus on the macro level, analysing statistics from the International Federation of Robotics on the deployment of industrial robots in various manufacturing processes in Asia and Australia between 1998 and 2010. They show that this region dominates in terms of the number of robotic units installed, with applications in handling and welding, especially in the automotive and electrical engineering industries, accounting for the lion's share. The study documents very well the trends in robot adoption and the differences between countries (Korea, Japan, China), but it remains at the statistical level – it does not evaluate qualitative changes in production or specific impacts on workplace layout or material flow [24]. Critically, although there is a relatively rich literature on robotics in implant surgery and 3D printing of dental implants, there is an almost complete lack of work that comprehensively describes a robotised production workplace specifically focused on the production of dental implants – with the interconnection of additive manufacturing, machining, quality control and handling in a single integrated system. Most of the available studies either focus on individual technological nodes (robots in surgery, 3D printing, surface treatment) or describe robotic cells in other industrial sectors. This identified research deficit supports the justification for conducting a simulation study of a robotic workplace for the production of dental implants and creates space for the design of a methodology that links knowledge from clinical implantology, additive manufacturing and industrial robotics.

3 Robotic Workplace Design for Additive Manufacturing of Dental Implants

As part of the practical section, a 3D model of a robotic workplace was created using Tecnomatix Plant Simulation software. The created workplace was also analysed during the simulation, and the graphs generated show the smooth progress of the work cycle. The workplace shown (see Fig. 3) represents a fully automated production cell designed for the additive manufacturing of dental implants. The entire system is enclosed by a safety fence with an entrance gate, which separates the operators from the automated equipment.

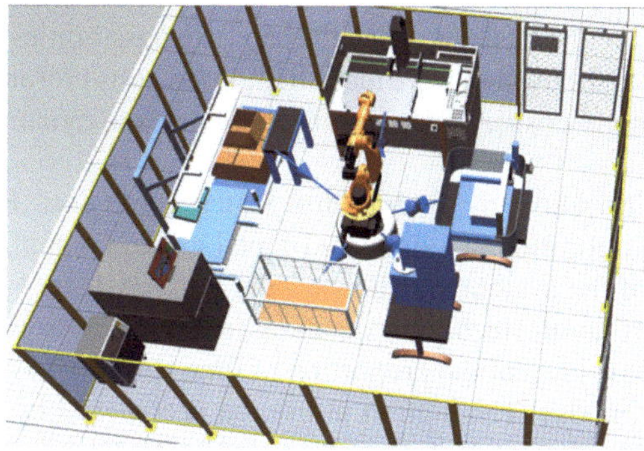

Fig. 3. Designed workplace using Tecnomatix Plant Simulation software.

The central element of the workplace is an industrial robot that handles parts between individual production and processing stations. The workplace consists of the following technological nodes:

At the rear of the cell is a 3D printer for metal materials, probably of the SLM/DMLS type, which produces titanium dental implants. The printer is equipped with:

- powder feeding systems,
- a control panel,
- a working platform for printing.

After completing the process, the robot removes the finished parts or the carrier with the manufactured series of implants.

Next to the printer is a workstation used for:

- removing residual metal powder,
- separating the implants from the support structures,
- initial mechanical processing.

The robot moves the parts here directly from the 3D printer.

On the right-hand side is a device for the final surface treatment of implants, which may include:

- sandblasting or shot blasting,
- vibration/abrasion treatment,
- micro-milling of seating surfaces,
- or surface chemical treatments (anodising, etching).

The workstation is equipped with a protective cover and handling devices.

Next to the robot is an output basket container into which the robot places the finished and inspected implants. The design allows entire containers to be removed without interrupting the cycle.

4 Results and Discussion

The workplace was analysed using simulation software, which enabled detailed monitoring of the behaviour of individual resources throughout the entire production process. During the simulation, operating conditions, time sequences and equipment utilisation levels were recorded, on the basis of which the capacity possibilities were evaluated and potential bottlenecks in the system were identified. The results presented in the following graphs provide a comprehensive picture of the efficiency and dynamics of the modelled workplace.

The Resource Utilisation by Operational States graph (see Fig. 4) provides an overview of resource utilisation in a simulated dental implant manufacturing workplace. The main elements of the system are shown – the PickAndPlace1 handling robot, the Station, Station1 and Station2 technology stations, and the Source parts input generator. The coloured sections represent the proportion of time spent on „Working", "Waiting", "Blocked" and other modes. The highest utilisation is achieved by the PickAndPlace1 robot, which works approximately 45% of the time, while the rest is spent waiting. The robot does not represent a bottleneck in the system, although more than 50% of the waiting time indicates the possibility of optimising the flow of parts. The main technological station (Station) only works about 20% of the time, with approximately 80% of the time spent waiting. Its capacity is therefore excessive and does not limit production throughput. The input source of parts (Source) is almost constantly in "Waiting" mode, which is due to its function – parts are generated only on demand for subsequent operations. Stations Station1 and Station2 exhibit similar behaviour: 22–25% working time, 70–72% waiting time and a small percentage of blockages (around 5%). These blockages are caused by the output space being full, but their extent is minimal. The results show that the technological operations are significantly underutilised and the system has a large capacity reserve. The graph confirms that the workplace is oversized in its current configuration and most of the equipment is operating at low capacity. There are no bottlenecks and production throughput is not limited by any station. The workplace is therefore capable of absorbing increased demand without expanding the technological units. At the same time, however, the high proportion of "Waiting" states indicates potential for optimising material flow, shortening handling times and improving coordination between the robot and operations, which could improve the overall efficiency of the workplace.

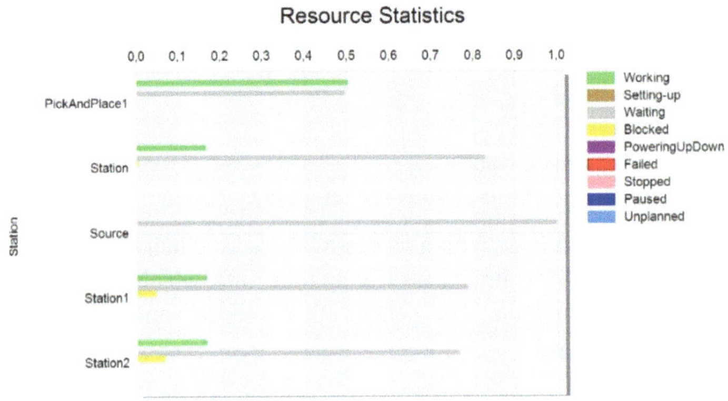

Fig. 4. Resource Utilisation by Operational States.

The graph Distribution of Operational States Across Resources (see Fig. 5) provides an overview of the time distribution of the states of individual workplace resources: PickAndPlace1, Station, Source, Station1, and Station2. Across all devices, the most dominant state identified is Waiting, in which most of the time is spent waiting for parts to arrive or for the next work step to be released. This behaviour indicates that the workplace is oversized in terms of capacity and no element of the system is overloaded. The PickAndPlace1 handling robot is assigned to the highest level of active work (Working), reaching approximately 45%, making it the busiest resource in the process. In contrast, the technological stations Station1 and Station2 are used for a shorter time; their active operation is supplemented by minimal blocking states (Blocked), which are caused by temporary filling of the output or input positions. These blockages are small in scope and are not considered significant flow constraints. The input source Source is practically exclusively in a waiting state, which is due to its function – parts are generated only as needed by the system. None of the stations show failure (Failed), stoppage (Stopped) or unplanned outages (Unplanned) states, confirming the stable operation of the modelled workplace. The overall graph shows that the workplace is stable in terms of production capacity, with no identified bottlenecks, and that processes run smoothly with significant time reserves for possible future increases in production.

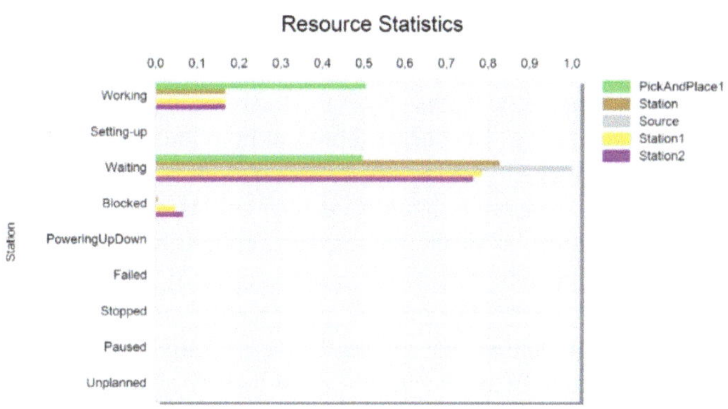

Fig. 5. Distribution of Operational States Across Resources.

The pie chart Dynamic Time Evolution of Resource Occupancy (see Fig. 6) shows the percentage distribution of active working time (Working) of individual workplace resources. The PickAndPlace1 handling robot is identified as having the largest share of active activity, accounting for more than 50.2% of all operations performed. This result confirms that it is the busiest element of the workplace and a key node in the operation of technological stations. The technological stations Station, Station1 and Station2 are assigned the same share of active work, approximately 16.6% for each, which indicates an even distribution of technological operations between these nodes. The Source and Drain are not included in the graph as they do not show any active working time; their zero share is consistent with their function of generating and removing parts without performing technological operations. The graph thus indicates that the workplace is designed with a dominant handling robot that performs most of the movement and handling tasks, while the technological stations contribute to the overall processing of parts with evenly distributed shares of active work.

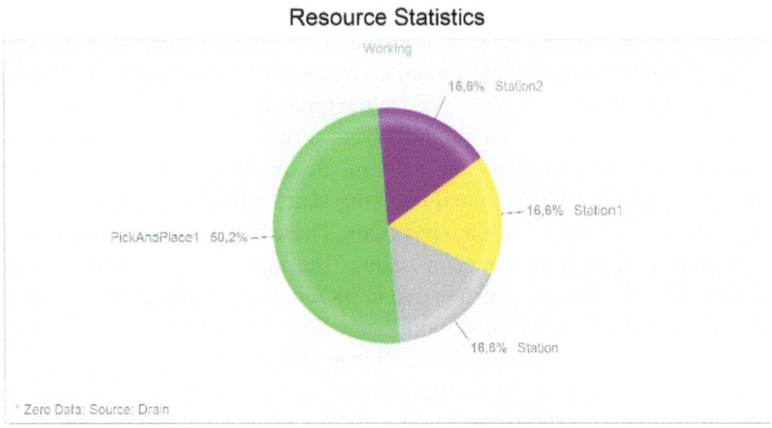

Fig. 6. Dynamic Time Evolution of Resource Occupancy.

The graph Temporal Progression of Resource Operational States (see Fig. 7) shows the time progression of the utilisation of individual resource states in the workplace during the simulation. The vertical axis shows the load level (0–1), while the horizontal axis shows the passage of time. The curves represent individual operational states, such as Working, Waiting, Blocked, Setting up, Failed, Stopped, Paused, and Unplanned. At the beginning of the simulation, significant fluctuations are observed in all states, which is caused by the start-up of the process, the initialisation of resources and the gradual stabilisation of the material flow. After approximately 30–40 min, the operating modes stabilise and the curves become stable. In steady state, Waiting is identified as the dominant state, indicating that resources – especially technological stations – are left in waiting mode most of the time for the arrival of parts or the completion of previous operations. This state reaches the highest values (approximately 0.6–0.7), which corresponds to the results of other graphs, which showed that the manipulator is the most utilised element of the workplace, while the remaining stations show lower operational utilisation. The Working state stabilises at a value of approximately 0.4, confirming that resources are actively working less than half the time, with the rest being downtime. Other states – Blocked, Setting-up, Stopped, Paused or Failed – occur only minimally and show very low values, which indicates high workplace stability and minimal occurrence of faults or the need to reconfigure equipment. The overall course of the graph shows that after the initial stabilization phase; the system enters an equilibrium mode in which the dominance of the "Waiting" and "Working" states is repeatedly confirmed. This indicates potential for optimisation, for example by reducing waiting times or balancing the workflow between stations more efficiently.

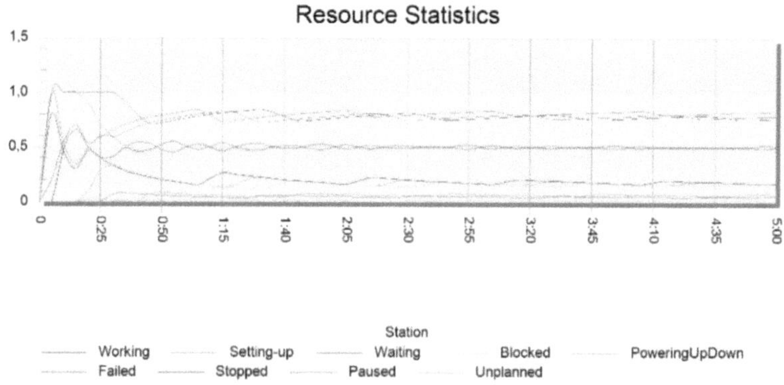

Fig. 7. Temporal Progression of Resource Operational States.

Graph 3D Visualisation of Resource Occupancy Versus Number of Manufacturing Units (see Fig. 8) shows the percentage utilisation of workplace resources depending on the number of manufacturing units (MUs) and the proportion of time during which individual resources are active. This is a spatial 3D graph that allows you to monitor changes in workplace occupancy at different levels of system load. The value on the vertical axis represents the percentage of time during which the resources were occupied (0–100%). The horizontal axis shows the number of MUs, i.e. the number of parts passing through the production system, and the third axis shows the time share that characterises the dynamics of resource utilisation during the simulation. The graph clearly shows that at low MU values, system utilisation is low, which means that resources are not fully utilized. As the number of parts increases, utilisation increases rapidly, and at approximately medium load, values of 50–100% are achieved, indicating optimal utilisation of workstations. At the maximum number of parts, a decrease in stability and increased variability in utilisation is observed, probably caused by capacity limits or the emergence of bottlenecks in the workflow. This variability points to the need to optimise the number of input parts to avoid overloading handling and production stations. Overall, the graph indicates that the highest workplace efficiency is achieved at medium production volumes, while too low or too high a load leads to underutilisation or, conversely, overloading of the system.

The Active Working Time Distribution Among Resources graph (see Fig. 9) shows the percentage utilization of individual workplace resources for different numbers of manufacturing units (MUs). The vertical axis shows the time share [%], which expresses how much of the simulation a given resource was active, while the horizontal axis shows the number of MUs (in this case 0 and 1), i.e. the number of parts processed in the system. At 0 MUs, it can be observed that most devices show very high utilisation at 90–100% (e.g. Conveyor, Conveyor2, Drain, Station1, Station2). This state is typical for the model initialisation phase, when resources are being set up, undergoing initial process operations or kept in a ready state without actively processing parts. Some elements, such as Conveyor1 and Source, show lower values (e.g., 80% or 45%), reflecting the shorter duration of their active phase in the initial part of the simulation. At 1 MU, there is a significant decrease in the utilisation of most equipment, with values ranging mainly

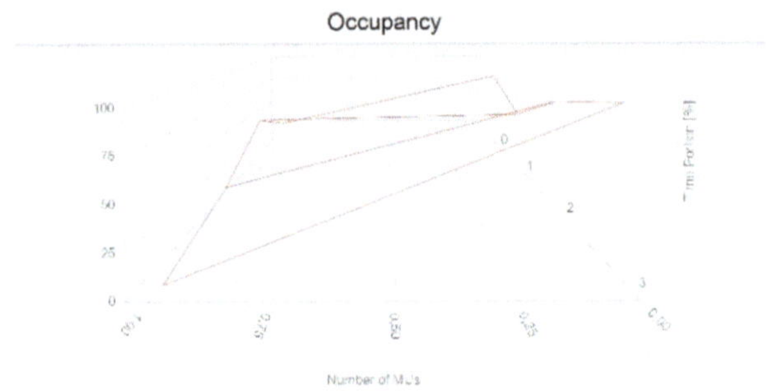

Fig. 8. 3D Visualisation of Resource Occupancy Versus Number of Manufacturing Units.

between 0–30%. This means that resources are not continuously loaded when processing a single part. The exception is the Source resource, which reaches approximately 58% at 1 MU, due to its function of ensuring the entry of parts into the system. Overall, the graph shows significant underutilisation of the system at low production load (1 MU), with individual stations operating only for short periods of time. Conversely, at zero load, some resources are kept at high occupancy due to initial setup or internal model processes. The graph allows the level of utilisation of individual workplace components to be identified under different simulation conditions.

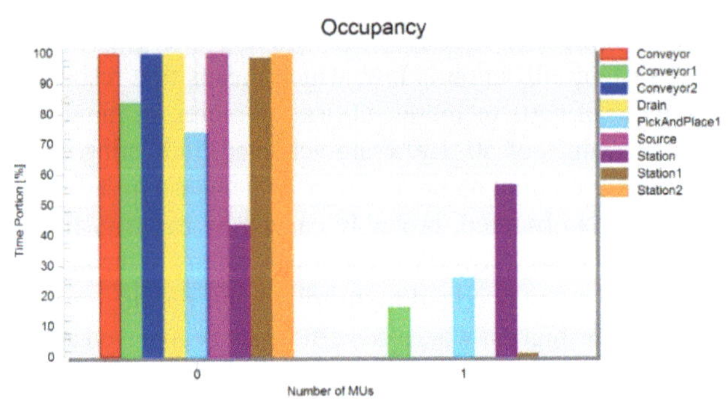

Fig. 9. Active Working Time Distribution Among Resources

The graph Visualisation of Resource Occupancy Versus Number of Manufacturing Units (see Fig. 10) shows the dynamic development of the utilisation of individual workplace resources over time during the processing of manufacturing units (MUs). The horizontal axis shows the simulation time, while the vertical axis shows the resource occupancy rate with values ranging from 0 to 1 (or slightly above 1, depending on the model normalisation method). Each curve represents one workplace resource – conveyors (Conveyor, Conveyor1, Conveyor2), cleaning and finishing stations (Station, Station1, Station2), robot PickAndPlace1, Source and Drain. The graph is characterised by cyclical oscillations resulting from repeated production operations. The sources are alternately found in a state of high utilisation (during part processing) and in a state of minimum utilisation (during waiting or transitions between operations). These cyclical waves show regularity, confirming the stable functioning of the production process at a constant rate. The graph shows that several resources repeatedly reach near-maximum utilisation (close to 1), particularly the PickAndPlace1 robot, conveyors and output stations. This indicates that these devices are key points in the production flow and are continuously involved in the process. Minor oscillations at some stations indicate short periods of inactivity caused by waiting times between operations or logistical transitions. The overall picture of the graph shows that the workplace is operated in a stable cyclic mode, in which individual resources are regularly involved in the process according to their production tasks. This type of visualisation also makes it possible to identify potential production bottlenecks – in particular, equipment that operates close to its maximum capacity for long periods of time and may represent a future limiting factor in performance.

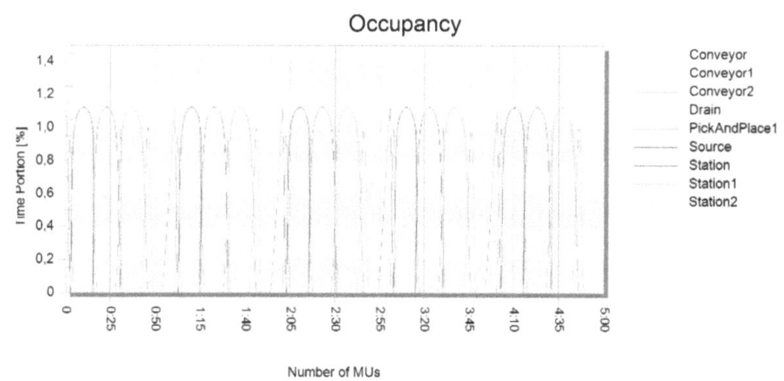

Fig. 10. 3D Visualisation of Resource Occupancy Versus Number of Manufacturing Units

5 Conclusion

The simulation study showed that the proposed robotic workplace for the production of dental implants is a functional and stable solution capable of ensuring a smooth production flow. The results of the analysis of the Resource Statistics, Occupancy and pie charts confirmed that the individual resources are operating without significant disruptions and that the system is entering a stable operating mode after the initial stabilisation phase. The dominance of the "Waiting" states indicated a high-capacity reserve of the equipment, while the utilisation of the "Working" state confirmed that the main production operations are evenly distributed among the technological stations. The industrial robot proved to be the most heavily loaded element of the workplace, reflecting its key role in the parts handling process. Analysis of resource utilisation under different production conditions showed that the system achieves maximum efficiency at medium production loads. With a low number of production units, the equipment was underutilised, while at maximum load, higher variability in utilisation was observed, which may lead to bottlenecks in the future. The simulation model thus provided valuable insights into workplace behaviour and identified potential areas for optimisation, in particular reducing waiting times and improving coordination between the robot and individual operations. The results confirm the validity of integrating industrial robots and additive manufacturing in the field of dental implants. The simulation also showed that appropriate material flow and workplace layout can significantly contribute to increasing its efficiency. The proposed model provides a basis for further optimisation studies and can serve as a basis for the real-world implementation of robotic workplaces in healthcare manufacturing.

Acknowledgements. This research was supported by the Scientific Grant Agency of the Ministry of Education, Research, Development and Youth of the Slovak Republic and Slovak Academy of Sciences, grant VEGA 1/0258/24. This work was supported by the Slovak Research and Development Agency under contract No. APVV-21-0293. Also, it was supported by project DRP0200194, Moving Plastics and Machine Industry towards Circularity (PLAN-C) under the Interreg Danube Region Program, co-funded by the European Union.

References

1. Glaser A (2008) Industrial robotics. Industrial Press, New York
2. Groover MP, Weiss M, Nagel RN (1986) Industrial robotics: technology, programming and application. McGraw-Hill Higher Education, New York
3. Beaverstock M, Greenwood A, Nordgren W (2018) Applied simulation: modeling and analysis using FlexSim. BookBaby, Scotts Valley, CA
4. Sharma P (2015) Discrete-event simulation. Int J Sci Technol Res 4(4):136–140
5. Chryssolouris G (2006) Manufacturing systems: theory and practice. Springer, New York, NY
6. Robinson S (2008) Conceptual modelling for simulation part I: definition and requirements. J Oper Res Soc 59(3):278–290
7. Vaisi B, Farughi H, Raissi S (2018) Two-machine robotic cell sequencing under different uncertainties. Int J Simul Model 17:284–294
8. Tran N-H, Park H-S, Nguyen Q-V, Hoang T-D (2019) Development of a smart cyber-physical manufacturing system in the industry 4.0 context. Appl Sci 9(16):3325
9. Semjon J et al (2020) Verification of the UR5 robot's properties after a crash caused by a fall of a transferred load from a crane. Int J Adv Robotic Syst 17(1):1729881420904209
10. Warreth A, Ibieyou N, O'Leary RB, Cremonese M, Abdulrahim M (2017) Dental implants: an overview. Dent Update 44(7):596–620
11. Silva M et al (2017) Application of a hybrid additive manufacturing methodology to produce a metal/polymer customised dental implant. Procedia Manuf 12:150–155
12. Gandhi P, Chaudhari N, Bhole K (2012) Fabrication of textured 3D micro-structures using bulk lithography. In: Proc. ASME Int. Manuf. Sci. Eng. Conf. (MSEC). Notre Dame, USA, pp 959–964
13. Kale BS, Bhole KS, Sharma C (2021) Effect of anisotropies in formation of viscous fingering in lifting plate hele–Shaw cell. Adv Mater Process Technol 8:3780. https://doi.org/10.1080/2374068X.2021.2013679
14. Ramakrishnaiah R et al (2017) Preliminary fabrication and characterisation of electron beam melted Ti–6Al–4V customised dental implant. Saudi J Biol Sci 24(4):787–796
15. Patil AS, Sunnapwar VK, Bhole KS, More YS (2021) Experimental investigation and fuzzy TOPSIS optimisation of Ti6Al4V finish milling. Adv Mater Process Technol 8:3706. https://doi.org/10.1080/2374068X.2021.1971002

16. Kasambe PV, Bhole KS, Bhoir DV (2021) Analytical modelling, design optimisation and numerical simulation of a variable width cantilever beam MEMS switch. Adv Mater Process Technol 8:1–21. https://doi.org/10.1080/2374068X.2021.1945263
17. Alqutaibi AY, Alghauli AM, Aljohani MHA, Zafar MS (2024) Advanced additive manufacturing in implant dentistry: 3D printing technologies, printable materials, current applications and future requirements. Bio-printing 42:e00356
18. Pradies G et al (2024) Current applications of 3D printing in dental implantology: a scoping review mapping the evidence. Clin Oral Implants Res 35(8):1011–1032
19. Chen Y, Wei J (2025) Application of 3D printing technology in dentistry: a review. Polymers 17(7):886
20. Montini E et al (2024) An industrial human–robot collaboration case study for workers' well-being. Procedia CIRP 130:924–929
21. Wang K, Ding L, Dailami F, Matthews J (2025) A contemporary review of collaborative robotics employed in manufacturing finishing operations: recent progress and future directions. Machines 13(9):772
22. Barosz P, Gołda G, Kampa A (2020) Efficiency analysis of manufacturing line with industrial robots and human operators. Appl Sci 10(8):2862
23. Makulavičius M et al (2023) Industrial robots in mechanical machining: perspectives and limitations. Robotics 12(6):160
24. Karabegović I, Karabegović E, Husak E (2013) Industrial robot applications in manufacturing processes in Asia and Australia. Tehnički vjesnik 20(2):365–370

Additive Manufacturing of Individualized Anatomical Models to Support Otolaryngologic Surgery Planning

Emilia Smolarek[1](✉), Dominik Kłak[1], Błażej Gabryszewski[1], Magdalena Żukowska[1], Filip Górski[1], and Anders Nøhr[2]

[1] Division of Additive Manufacturing and Virtual Reality, Poznan University of Technology, Poznan, Poland
emilia.smolarek@doctorate.put.poznan.pl

[2] Department of Otorhinolaryngology, Head and Neck Surgery and Audiology, Rigshospitalet, Copenhagen, Denmark

Abstract. This study presents the potential of additive manufacturing for creating patient-specific anatomical models to support surgical planning in complex cases. Two approaches were investigated: PolyJet technology, enabling the production of uniform, multi-material, and multi-color models with high-quality visualization of anatomical structures and precise tissue differentiation and a combination of DLP printing with vacuum casting, offering a more cost-effective alternative that provides realistic tactile properties and the possibility of presenting cross-sections of critical structures. Expert evaluation confirmed the usefulness of both methods in understanding spatial relationships, enhancing team communication, and supporting surgical preparation. Economic analysis revealed significant differences in material costs and production time, highlighting the importance of a deliberate choice of technology and materials depending on the desired balance between accuracy, functionality, and cost. The study demonstrates that patient-specific anatomical models are valuable tools for surgical planning and personalized medicine, requiring close collaboration between clinical and engineering teams to ensure both anatomical precision and practical usability.

Keywords: Additive Manufacturing · Anatomical Models · Surgical Planning

1 Introduction

1.1 An Introduction

The development of modern oncology emphasizes the need for use of advanced technologies in surgical planning. Traditionally preoperative decisions were based on standard medical imaging, clinical assessment and experience of the operating team [1]. However, with increasing complexity of oncological cases and demand of minimizing risk of complications, this approach does does not provide sufficient solutions [2, 3]. In this context the importance of pre-surgery models increases.

F. Górski et al. (Eds.): MANUFACTURING 2026, LNME, pp. 70–84, 2026.
https://doi.org/10.1007/978-3-032-23089-8_7

Pre-surgery models are focused on delivering precise information about a patient's anatomy and occurring pathologies, and in cancer cases about tumor characteristics, its biology and operative risk as well as its localization and tumor extent [4–6]. They form a foundation of personalized medicine whose fundamental premise is to tailor therapeutic processes to unique needs and characteristics of a patient. They integrate clinical data, medical imaging and recently even very specific parameters and artificial intelligence, helping medical professionals in tailoring surgical strategy to individual characteristics of a patient's case [3, 7, 8]. The requirements for surgery models are determined by the team of experienced team of medical professionals who undertake the specific procedure which patients will undergo. During specifying these requirements it's crucial to take into consideration a function the model is supposed to fill. The main roles that individualized model can play are: simulation, visualization and tooling. The simulation function can help the doctors to plan the surgical approach and theories [9] and the visual function is to familiarise with the patients case and anatomical relations between structures as well as enabling the proper communication with the patient. The tool function allows for the individualization of medical procedures, which are based on specific patient's anatomy and characteristics. One of the most important challenges of preparing pre-surgery models for cancer cases is taking both tumor biology and anatomical factors, which determine the safety of the procedure [10]. Additionally additive manufacturing enables for structures to have complex geometries, not achievable by traditional manufacturing methods, while being faster at the same time [11, 12]. In complicated cases with difficult surgical access such as tumors localised near the spinal cord [13] or close to the big blood vessels [14] or even in cases of extensive fractures (Fig. 1) use of only medical imaging may not be sufficient for predicting full resection range or need for reconstructive surgeries [6]. In these cases 3D printed models help surgeons to better plan the surgical access and predict complications.

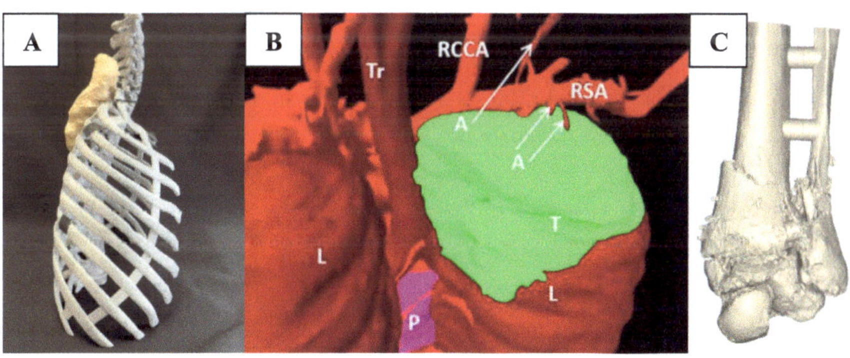

Fig. 1. Preoperative models of (A) spinal column tumor [13] (B) thoracic tumor [14] (C) femoral fracture [6].

Additive manufacturing can be divided in three main categories: rapid prototyping, rapid manufacturing and rapid tooling. Rapid prototyping is used for creating models and prototypes, which are not final products but replicas of manufactured products used for validating the project when still in development and for optimizing the process of manufacturing such as vents for rail vehicles [15]. Rapid manufacturing method can be used to obtain parts of the final product and even the product itself e. g. cover for cable routing in aircrafts [16]. Rapid tooling is used to create tools that are meant to be produced in small quantities and in a short time for example molds in injection molding [17].

Additive manufacturing is becoming increasingly popular in many fields of medicine such as surgery, farmacology production and testing as well as bioprinting. Adjusting the parameters of printing as well as appropriate choice of manufacturing method can prove useful creating not only visual and educational models but create implants and surgical guides with specific properties and even complicated shapes.

The use of pre - surgery models is particularly important in cases of tumors with difficult biological characteristics, fast growing tumors and high bleeding risk [14]. In these types of cases the models can help in predicting the resection margin and also tell if the reconstruction will be needed, while helping the surgical team to prepare for possible post-surgery complications [18]. However, despite huge growth pre-surgery models still face numerous problems including cost, scalability and standardization as well as limited selection of the materials available as they need to mimic the feel and mechanical properties of actual human tissue [11, 19]. Additionally the quality of imaging which models are based on is variable and depends on the used equipment, examination protocol and experience of the radiologist [20]. The abilities and experience of the engineer preparing the models are also one of the factors that affects the quality of the model. Personalized medicine sees each patient as the individual, who has to be treated in a specific way tailored to their own needs. Preoperative models allow for assessing which treatment strategy would be the most successful in threatening the specific patient [21]. Integrating the clinical data with the patient specific, 3D printed models can lead to better treatment response and identification of the areas with increased surgical risk (Fig. 2) [22].

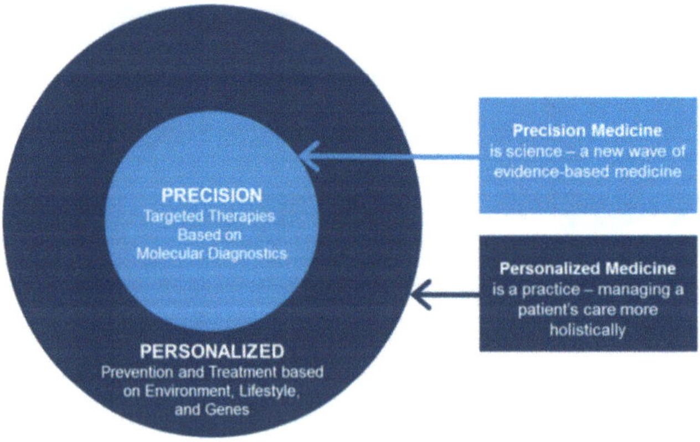

Fig. 2. Personalized and precision medicine [23].

2 Research Problem

Surgical procedures at the skull base are highly challenging due to the proximity of structures critical for auditory and vascular functions. In this study, we analyzed a patient case involving a tumor located in the region of the tympanic cavity and jugular vein, characteristic of a disease entity known as jugulotympanic paraganglioma (glomus tumor). Lesions of this type may remain in very close spatial relation with the internal carotid artery, internal jugular vein, and inner ear structures, which increases the risk of intraoperative complications, particularly massive bleeding. Due to the anatomical complexity of this region, such cases require collaboration between otolaryngology and neurosurgery teams, and the interpretation of CT and MRI imaging data does not always allow for a complete understanding of the three-dimensional configuration of structures relevant for surgical approach planning.

For this reason, the need was identified for the development of a patient-specific anatomical model, produced using high-resolution additive manufacturing technologies, capable of faithfully reproducing the patient's anatomy and meeting the clinicians' requirements for preoperative visualization of critical structures. From an engineering perspective, it was crucial to determine which additive manufacturing technologies and material configurations would enable the production of multi-material and multi-color models with high fidelity, while simultaneously providing functional properties that allow spatial analysis of planned surgical approaches.

3 Methodology

Analyzing the described case, two complementary approaches were employed, which highlight the complexity of the examined anatomy in different ways and allow the production of models with distinct material and functional properties (Fig. 3). Both approaches ensured high model accuracy and met the requirements for differentiating hardness and transparency of anatomical structures.

The first method utilized PolyJet technology, in which liquid photopolymer resins are deposited as microscopic droplets layer by layer and cured with UV light, allowing precise multi-material and multi-color fabrication. This technology is characterized by high resolution and smooth surface finish, and the use of multiple materials enables the creation of multi-material, multi-color models produced within a single manufacturing process, in which individual components differ in hardness and transparency. The second approach involved DLP (Digital Light Processing) technology, where photopolymers contained in a resin vat are cured with UV projector light. DLP provides high detail reproduction of fine anatomical structures at a relatively low manufacturing cost. To enhance the model's functionality, additional silicone casts were incorporated, allowing for soft elements that mimic tissue properties. Prior to manufacturing, anatomical structures were segmented based on CT and MRI data provided by the clinical team. These segmentations served as the basis for preparing models for both printing technologies:

- The PolyJet model included the temporal bone, internal carotid artery and vein, cochlea, semicircular canals, vestibulocochlear nerve, and tumor. The model was produced as a single, unified structure, enabling detailed visualization of the spatial relationships between anatomical components.

- The DLP model comprised the temporal bone divided into two parts and the internal carotid artery. The model was complemented with a silicone tumor, allowing the inclusion of flexible elements.

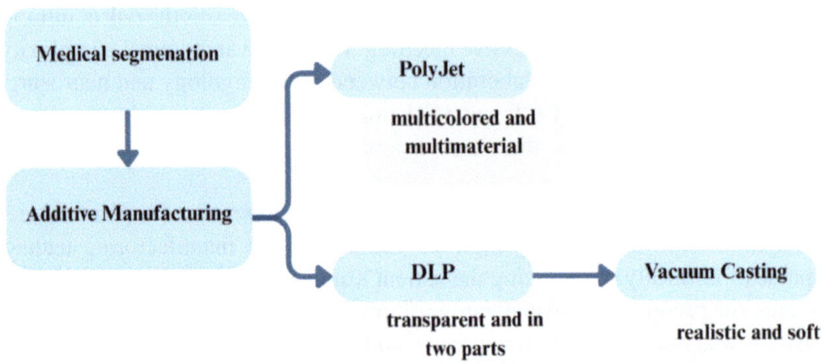

Fig. 3. Concept for additive manufacturing of patient-specific craniofacial models.

3.1 PolyJet Additive Manufacturing

The manufacturing workflow began with the PolyJet process. PolyJet technology was used to produce a single transparent model with internal anatomical structures represented in different colors. Model preparation for fabrication was carried out in GrabCAD Print. The PolyJet manufacturing procedure involved assigning selected materials and colors to the individual components of the model and correctly positioning the object on the build platform. An important aspect was orienting the model so that the key structures, those whose visibility is essential for the surgical perspective, were not supported (Fig. 4). This is due to surface hazing caused by the support material adhering to the walls. Incorrect orientation on the build platform could limit the visibility of the tumor and adjacent structures, lower the quality and functionality of the model, and increase cleaning time because additional surface finishing would be required.

The model, consisting of six elements, was imported as an assembly, which allowed the phantom to be produced as a whole with properly aligned structures embedded in the bone component. Each element was assigned a color based on combinations of primary, hard resins. Blood vessels were colored red and blue, the nerve yellow, the inner ear structures green, and the tumor in shades of brown. The only exception was the bone component, which was assigned a transparent material to allow visualization of the internal structures. The estimated manufacturing time was 5 h 47 min (Fig. 5). The device settings include a system-defined exposure time to UV light and a constant layer thickness of 0.018 mm.

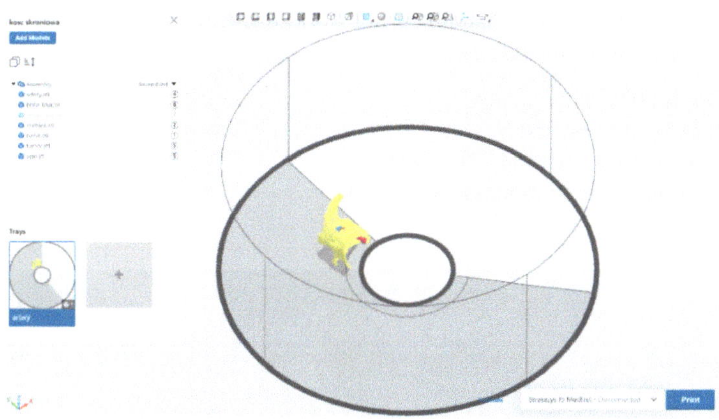

Fig. 4. View of the correctly positioned model on the build platform.

Print Time	5h 47m
Total Materials (g)	103
Total Support (g)	79
DraftWhite (g)	28
ElasticoClear (g)	62
VeroCyan-V (g)	4
VeroMagenta-V (g)	4
VeroYellow-V (g)	5
SUP710 (g)	79

Fig. 5. Estimation of manufacturing time and material consumption.

The final product required removal of the support material in a pressurized water chamber. The model was first cleaned with a stronger water jet, and then precision cleaning was used to remove excess material from holes and narrow areas. Final cleaning was carried out outside the chamber using a scalpel and a needle to remove supports adhering directly to the walls of the product and to clear hard-to-reach areas.

3.2 DLP Additive Manufacturing

For the production of the modular model using DLP technology, a Phrozen Sonic Mini 8 K printer was used, providing high resolution and precise reproduction of fine anatomical structures. A transparent photopolymer resin was selected, enabling the creation of transparent model elements that allowed visualization of the internal bone structure and facilitated subsequent integration with a silicone cast representing the tumor. Model preparation for additive manufacturing was performed in Chitubox 1.9.5 software, where the spatial orientation of the components was defined and a support system was added. Proper support design is critical in DLP technology, as it prevents model deformation and minimizes the risk of detachment from the build platform during printing (Fig. 6).

During the preparation of the manufacturing workflow, exposure parameters and layer structures were defined, including:

- Layer height: 0,05 mm
- Number of bottom layers: 6
- Bottom layer exposure time: 35 s
- Exposure time for remaining layers: 10,5 s.

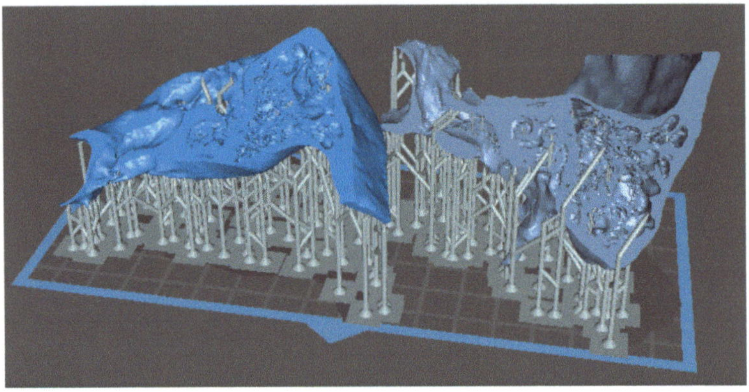

Fig. 6. View of the models with supports arranged on the build platform.

In the final stage of data preparation, the model was converted into a set of slices, which is a standard procedure in DLP technology. This process involves dividing the 3D geometry into a sequence of two-dimensional cross-sections corresponding to successive layers of cured photopolymer. Before printing, the photopolymer resin was thoroughly mixed to ensure complete homogenization of all its components. After printing, post-processing was performed. The first step involved washing the model in isopropyl alcohol (IPA) using a dedicated device to remove any uncured resin from the surface. For the model described, the washing time was set to 10 min. After washing, the support structures were manually removed. The model was then cured under UV light, which stabilized the surface and strengthened the structures prior to final support removal, a process requiring precision and care due to delicate details. The UV exposure time was set to 10 min.

3.3 Vacuum Casting

The final manufacturing technique employed in this study was vacuum casting, used to produce a realistic representation of the tumor. Vacuum casting was a key step in producing the model containing a realistic tumor. The process began with the design of a two-part casting mold in 3D Builder, which allowed for easy separation of the mold halves and precise positioning of the internal components. During the design process, Boolean operations (union, subtract, intersect) were applied to accurately define the space for the cast, generate mold cavities, and create guides ensuring stable and reproducible alignment of both mold halves.

A 6 mm pouring hole was created in the upper part of the mold, positioned in the area with the simplest geometry. This minimized the visibility of the pouring channel in the final cast, increased anatomical realism, and facilitated the introduction of higher-viscosity silicone. The final mold design was saved in STL format (Fig. 7) and prepared for additive manufacturing using FDM (Fused Deposition Modeling). Printing was performed on a Bambu Lab P1S printer using PLA filament, with the following parameters:

- Layer height: 0,20 mm
- Number of walls: 6
- Infill density: 10%.

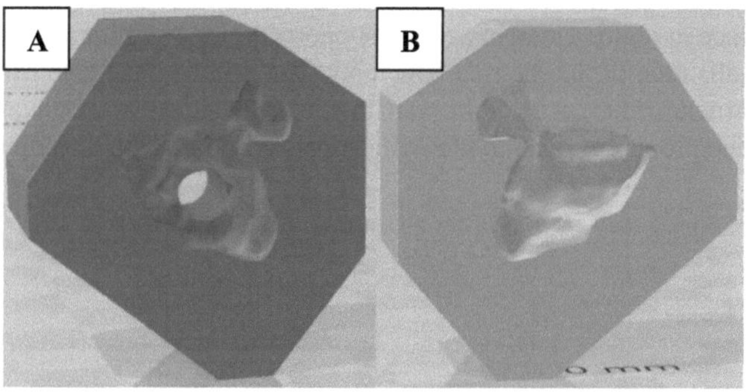

Fig. 7. Final mold.

For casting, Sorta Clear 37 addition-cure silicone was used. Material selection was based on literature analysis and previous team experience. The silicone was prepared in a 1:1 ratio of base and activator, yielding a 5 g mixture. To enhance realism, a small amount of brown Silc Pig pigment was added, which also facilitated tumor identification among other anatomical structures.

Before filling the mold, the silicone mixture was degassed in a vacuum chamber to remove air bubbles and significantly improve surface quality. After degassing, the silicone was poured into the mold through the pouring hole. The filled mold was placed again in the vacuum chamber to ensure uniform filling and eliminate remaining air bubbles. The silicone's working time of 25 min allowed precise filling of the entire mold cavity. The material was then left to fully cure for 4 h, in accordance with the manufacturer's instructions and material properties. After curing, the mold halves were separated, and any small excess silicone at the pouring channel was removed with a scalpel. This final operation ensured a smooth surface finish while maintaining a high level of anatomical realism in the model.

4 Results

4.1 Additive Manufacturing

All models achieved satisfactory surface quality. To obtain a transparent model using PolyJet technology, Elastico Clear material was used. The remaining structures in this model were printed with Draft White material, with different colors applied to facilitate identification of individual structures and to distinguish them from the bone. Relatively bright colors were chosen to enhance visibility. The printing process proceeded without issues. Support removal from the external surfaces of the model was not problematic. However, removing supports automatically generated by the software inside narrow openings, such as the ear canal, proved more challenging. This required the use of delicate, narrow tools, and even needles, to reach difficult-to-access areas. In the transparent bone, the surface in regions in contact with supports became significantly matte, which hindered visualization of the internal structures. The printed bone also exhibited a relatively soft structure due to the thin wall thickness, which was disadvantageous for simulating bone properties. The model with supports and after their removal is shown in Fig. 8.

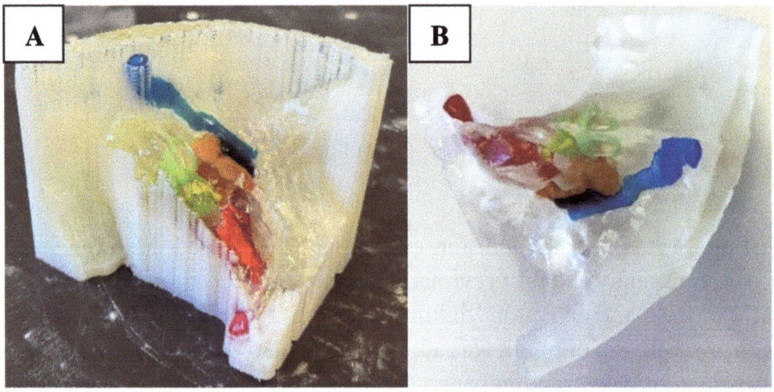

Fig. 8. PolyJet model: (A) with supports, (B) final model after support removal.

The DLP printing process was successful on the first attempt. The model was dimensionally accurate, and the two parts of the bone fitted together precisely. Post-processing proceeded smoothly: the supports detached easily and did not leave significant marks on the surface, owing to their appropriate placement during print preparation. The high resolution of the DLP technology enabled the reproduction of even fine anatomical details, including the mastoid air cells. Moreover, the sectional nature of the model allowed for a clear presentation of the spatial relationships between structures located adjacent to the tumor, such as the cochlea and the internal carotid artery (Fig. 9). The cured material exhibited suitable hardness, closely resembling the mechanical properties of bone tissue.

The silicone casting process for the tumor model was carried out twice. The first cast contained air bubbles in two areas, resulting in material voids and a reduction in both aesthetic quality and structural integrity. The second attempt was successful, producing

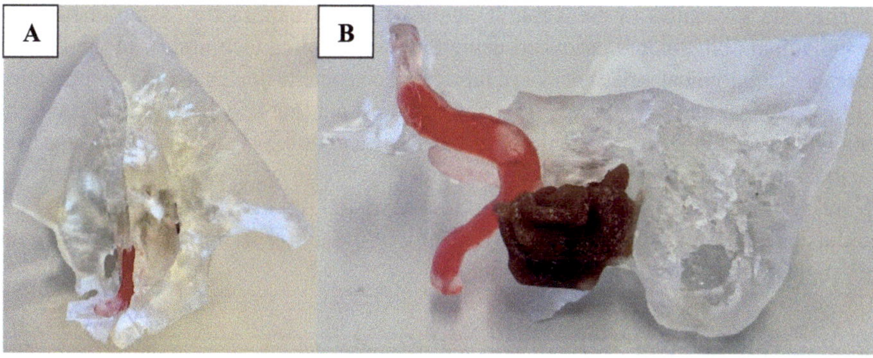

Fig. 9. DLP model: (A) assembled, inferior view; (B) cross-section showing the tumor and internal carotid artery.

a homogeneous structure free of air inclusions, with a smooth surface accurately replicating the anatomical geometry. The addition of a small amount of pigment enhanced the realism of the model (Fig. 9). The final cast exhibited elasticity similar to the palpation properties of real neoplastic tissue, indicating a high level of material fidelity.

Table 1. Summary of manufacturing of patient-specific craniofacial models.

Model	Material	Color	Printer	Manufacturing time
PolyJet				
Temporal bone	Elastico Clear	Transparent	Stratasys J5 MediJet	5 h 47 min
Internal carotid artery	Draft White VeroMagneta VeroCyan VeroYellow	Pink		
Internal jugular vein		Blue		
Cochlea		Green		
Semicircular canals		Green		
Vestibulocochlear nerve		Yellow		
Tumor		Brown		
DLP				
Temporal bone	Phrozen Aqua Clear	Transparent	Phrozen Sonic Mini 8 K	6 h 45 min
Vacuum Casting				
Mold	PLA	White	Bambu Lab P1S	37 min
Tumor	Sorta Clear 37 + Silc Pig pigment	Brown	–	4 h 30 min

The data presented in the Table 1 summarize the manufacturing parameters for the individual components produced using the three applied techniques. In the PolyJet process, all anatomical structures were fabricated on a single device using a combination of Elastico Clear and basic resins in various colors, enabling one-step production of the complete model in 5 h and 47 min. In the DLP technology, the temporal bone was manufactured from transparent Phrozen Aqua Clear resin with a total printing time of 6 h and 45 min. The silicone casting workflow involved separate fabrication of the PLA mold using FDM (37 min) followed by casting of the tumor in Sorta Clear 37 silicone with pigment, requiring 4 h and 30 min.

4.2 Expert Evaluation

To evaluate the models, a Likert-scale questionnaire was prepared, where 1 corresponded to "strongly disagree" and 5 to "strongly agree." The survey was administered separately for the PolyJet model and for the DLP + Vacuum Casting model, and it additionally included open-ended questions allowing experts to provide detailed comments. The questionnaire assessed, among other aspects, the accuracy of bone and soft-tissue representation, surface quality, clarity of anatomical details (e.g., blood vessels, nerves), material transparency, and the visibility of boundaries between structures. Experts also evaluated the usefulness of the models for understanding anatomical relationships, team communication, and their impact on confidence and precision during surgical planning.

The questionnaire was completed by two specialists with different clinical backgrounds, a neuroradiologist and a neurosurgeon, providing complementary perspectives on the utility of the 3D models. Both experts highly rated the representation of the bony structures, the tumor, as well as the semicircular canals and the cochlea in both the PolyJet and resin-based models (average scores: bone 4,5, tumor 5, semicircular canals 5, cochlea 5). They also agreed that the surface quality and clarity of details were generally satisfactory (surface quality 4, detail clarity 3,5) and that the models supported understanding of anatomical relationships (4,5) and facilitated team communication (4).

In several aspects, however, clear differences emerged between the experts. The neuroradiologist noted good visualization of blood vessels and nerves, whereas the neurosurgeon stated that the nerves were not visible enough to be useful for surgical planning. Similarly, the representation of mastoid air cells and arteries in the DLP model was rated highly by the neuroradiologist but as less clear by the neurosurgeon.

Both experts agreed that the models can support preoperative preparation, although the impact on surgical confidence and planning precision was rated as moderate (average score 2). They emphasized different elements they found most valuable: the neuroradiologist generally praised the use of the PolyJet technology, while the neurosurgeon appreciated the ability to inspect the tumor and its spatial relationships from multiple angles. Both suggested improving nerve visibility as the most critical enhancement for future iterations.

4.3 Economic Analysis

Table 2 presents a comparison of the key manufacturing parameters for 3D models produced using four different technologies: PolyJet, DLP, FDM, and vacuum casting.

The table includes model mass, manufacturing time, operator labor time, and material costs.

Table 2. Summary of key information on the produced models.

Model	PolyJet	DLP	FDM	Vaccum Casting
Mass [g]	103	62	19	5
Manufacturing time	5 h 47 min	6 h 45 min	37 min	4 h 30 min
Labor time	1 h 30 min	1 h	25 min	40 min
Cost [USD]	**890**	**5**	**8**	**11**
		24		

The model produced using PolyJet was fabricated in a single additive manufacturing process, whereas the second model involved a combination of multiple production processes, including DLP printing and silicone casting. Even after summing the masses of all components produced using DLP and silicone casting, the total mass (86 g) remained lower than that of the PolyJet model, which was 103 g.

The manufacturing time for the multi-material PolyJet model was relatively short. For the model produced using DLP, printing of the temporal bone required slightly more time, however, the silicone tumor casting was performed concurrently. The casting process itself was straightforward, with the longest stage being the complete polymerization of the material, which required approximately 4 h.

Material costs varied significantly across the technologies: the highest costs were associated with PolyJet (USD 890), while DLP required only USD 5. FDM printing incurred USD 8, and vacuum casting USD 11. These costs reflect only the expenses for machine operation and material consumption and do not account for design work or commercial margins, so they should be considered non-commercial estimates.

5 Discussion

The conducted study demonstrated that each of the applied technologies possesses both advantages and limitations in the production of individualized anatomical models. The two main approaches, PolyJet technology and the combination of DLP printing with vacuum silicone casting, showed complementary capabilities in reproducing complex anatomical structures while providing functional realism for preoperative planning.

PolyJet technology enabled the fabrication of a single, multi-material, and multi-color model within a single additive manufacturing process. The use of different colors allowed for precise differentiation of individual anatomical structures, including internal components such as the cochlea and semicircular canals. Additionally, this technology allowed for variation in material properties, supporting the visualization of both hard and soft tissues within a single model. However, the Elastico Clear material, used in small, thin-walled elements of the temporal bone, proved relatively soft, limiting the simulation of real bone proper-ties. The PolyJet model had the highest mass (103 g) and material costs (USD 890), yet its production was relatively straightforward, requiring only a single printing procedure and a moderate operator labor time. The most time-consuming and demanding step was the removal of supports from narrow channels, with localized surface matting in areas of support contact hindering visualization of internal structures and spatial relationships.

In contrast, the approach based on DLP technology combined with silicone ca-sting involved multiple production stages: high-resolution printing of the tempo-ral bone and silicone casting of the tumor. The total mass of the model (67 g) along with the mold (19 g) was lower than that of the PolyJet model, and material costs were significantly reduced (USD 5 for DLP printing, USD 11 for silicone casting, and USD 8 for the FDM mold). Although DLP printing of the bone took slightly longer (6 h 45 min), the tumor casting could be performed simultaneously, optimizing the overall production time. The casting process itself was simple and fast, and because silicone does not bond with other materials, it was possible to use molds printed in FDM technology with PLA.

Expert evaluations indicated that both approaches supported preoperative preparation, including the understanding of spatial relationships between structures and team communication. Differences in the perceived utility of the models stemmed from distinct clinical needs: PolyJet provided superior color-based visualization of structures, whereas DLP combined with silicone casting offered realistic tactile properties and clear sectional representation.

Comparative analysis demonstrated distinct differences between the technologies. PolyJet provides high precision and multi-material, multi-color capabilities at higher cost, whereas DLP combined with silicone casting offers a more economical solution with sufficient accuracy and realistic soft-tissue representation, with FDM serving as a fast and low-cost method for mold fabrication. Overall, the choice of technology affects model fidelity, production time, labor, and cost. From a standardization and scalability perspective, the proposed workflow can be readily integrated into clinical practice using standard CT/MRI data and widely available additive manufacturing technologies; however, case-specific anatomical complexity may require substantial effort and close engineer–radiologist collaboration, despite the significant clinical value of physical 3D models.

6 Conclusions

This study presents the potential of additive manufacturing in creating individualized anatomical models that support surgical planning in complex clinical cases. Two approaches were proposed. PolyJet technology enabled the production of a single, multi-material, multi-color model with excellent visualization of anatomical structures, while the combination of DLP printing with vacuum casting provided a more economical alternative, offering realistic tactile properties and the ability to present cross-sections.

Expert evaluation confirmed that both approaches improve understanding of spatial relationships and support team communication, with differences reflecting specific clinical needs. Economic analysis highlighted significant cost differences, emphasizing the need to select technologies and materials while balancing accuracy, functionality, and cost.

In conclusion, individualized anatomical models represent a valuable tool for surgical planning and the advancement of personalized medicine. Achieving optimal outcomes requires careful selection of additive manufacturing technologies and close collaboration between clinical and engineering teams, ensuring that the models meet both anatomical accuracy and practical usability requirements.

Acknowledgments. The studies were realized with support provided by the BIOMEDIX project (Project No. 2024-1-LV01-KA220-HED-000255929), realized within the Erasmus+ programme.

References

1. Graves M (2013) The value of preoperative planning. J Orthop Trauma 27:S30–S34
2. Lyuksemburrg V, Abou-Hanna J et al (2023) Virtual reality for preoperative planning in complex surgical oncology: a single-center experience. J Surg Res 291:546–556
3. Chuen Wong K, Yan Sun E et al (2023) Mixed reality improves 3d visualization and spatial awareness of bone tumors for surgical planning in orthopaedic oncology: a proof of concept study. Orthop Res Rev 15:139–149
4. Ganguli A, Pagan-Diaz GJ et al (2018) 3D printing for preoperative planning and surgical training: a review. Biomed Microdevices 20:65
5. Punyaratabanhu T, Liacouras PC, Pairojboriboon S (2018) Using 3D models in orthopedic oncology: presenting personalized advantages in surgical planning and intraoperative outcomes. 3D Print Med 4:12
6. Paxton NC, Wilkinson BG et al (2023) Technical improvements in preparing 3D printed anatomical models for comminuted fracture preoperative planning. 3D print Med 9:25
7. Wang J et al (2024) Artificial intelligence assisted preoperative planning and 3D-printing guiding frame for percutaneous screw reconstruction in periacetabular metastatic cancer patients. Front Bioeng Biotechnol 12:1404937
8. Górski F et al (2025) Digitization & processing of anatomical data of biomedical products. In: BIOMEDIX: advancing biomedical innovation through digital transformation. Zenodo
9. Smolarek E, Górski F, Żukowska M, Słowik Ł, Okła M (2025) Partial maxillofacial reconstruction: design and additive manufacturing of individualized pre-and mid-surgery supplies. Adv Sci Technol Res J 19(8):114–125
10. Witowski JS, Pędziwiatr M, Major P, Budzyński A (2017) Cost-effective, personalized, 3D-printed liver model for preoperative planning before laparoscopic liver hemihepatectomy for colorectal cancer metastases. Int J Comput Assist Radiol Surg 12:2047–2054
11. Alzoubi L, Alijabali AAA, Tambuwala MM (2023) Empowering precision medicine: the impact of 3D printing on personalized therapeutic. AAPS PharmSciTech 24:228
12. Razvan P et al (2025) Additive manufacturing processes of innovative biomedical products. In: BIOMEDIX: advancing biomedical innovation through digital transformation. Zenodo
13. Mikula AL, Rhines LD et al (2025) Utility of 3D-printed models in the surgical planning for primary spine tumors: a survey of international spinal oncology experts. Global Spine J 15(4):2004–2013
14. Tan D, Yao J, Hua X et al (2020) Application of 3D modeling and printing technology in accurate resection of complicated thoracic tumors. Ann Transl Med 8(21):1342
15. Franowski M, Cichoński Z, Stępniewski Ł, Sawczuk W (2024) The use of 3D printing technology in prototypes of selected components for civil and military rail vehicles. Systemy Logistyczne Wojsk 61:129–146

16. Engineering.com. Airbus Takes on Stratasys 3D Printing for Serial Part Production. Last accessed 19 Nov 2025
17. Noble J, Walczak K, Dornfeld D (2014) Rapid tooling injection molded prototypes: a case study in artificial photosynthesis technology. Procedia CIRP 14:251–256
18. Fletcher J, Miskovic D (2020) Digital and 3D printed models for surgical planning. In: Digital surgery, pp 95–110
19. Spałek MJ, Bochyńska A et al (2016) Challenges and solutions in 3D printing for oncology: a narrative review. Chin Clin Oncol 13(4):49
20. Chow LS, Paramesran R (2016) Review of medical image quality assessment. Biomed Signal Process Control 27:145–154
21. Topol EJ (2014) Individualized medicine from prewomb to tomb. Cell 157(1):241–253
22. Lambin P, Rios-Velazquez E et al (2012) Radiomics: extracting more information from medical images using advanced feature analysis. Eur J Cancer 48:441–446
23. Glady G (2019) The bio immune(G)ene medicine or how to use a maximum of molecular resources of the cell for therapeutic purposes. Edelweiss Appl Sci Technol 3(1):26–29

Patient-Specific Implants, Prostheses, and Orthotic Devices

Research on Structural Design of Mechanically Decoupled Breast Implants Made by Fused Deposition Modeling Technology

Răzvan Păcurar[1], Cristina Ludusan[1](✉), Dolores Ojados[2], Joaquin Roca-González[2], Emilia Sabau[1], Cristina Borzan[1], Cristian Vilău[1], and Ancuţa Păcurar[1](✉)

[1] Technical University of Cluj-Napoca, Cluj-Napoca, Romania
cristina.ludusan@yahoo.com, ancuta.costea@tcm.utcluj.ro
[2] Polytechnic University of Cartagena, Cartagena, Spain

Abstract. This paper presents a breast implant designed as a mechanically decoupled system composed of external and internal structures. Fused Deposition Modeling (FDM) technology was considered for the experiments in combination with medical grade materials. The external circular, multi-arched structure has been designed in such way to ensure load absorption. MRI scans were processed in Slicer3D and SolidWorks to create three implant models, being subsequently analyzed through finite element simulations and compression tests made under a 30 N load for estimating its mechanical behavior. The outer structure was fabricated from thermoplastic polyurethane (TPU 85A) material with helical channels testing it using two types of FDM printers of fabricating of the complex structures designed in this way with specifically mechanical characteristics that are required for such type of implants.

Keywords: breast implant · fused deposition modeling · TPU 85A · finite element analysis · mechanical testing

1 Introduction

Additive Manufacturing (AM) has emerged as a transformative approach in biomedical engineering, enabling the fabrication of patient-specific implants with complex geometries and controlled mechanical properties [1]. Among the available AM methods, Fused Deposition Modeling (FDM) allow precise control over structural features such as designed geometries with specific infill density, providing the capability to customize mechanical behavior to the functional requirements of breast implants [2, 3]. This method is particularly suitable for breast implants, where specific mechanical characteristics required like elasticity to be reached out are critical [4]. Breast tissue as a whole presents a complex hierarchical structure, consisting of skin, fatty tissue, glandular tissue, fibrous ligaments, and muscles, each contributing to its mechanical response under static and dynamic loading [5]. These properties are strongly influenced by factors

F. Górski et al. (Eds.): MANUFACTURING 2026, LNME, pp. 87–99, 2026.
https://doi.org/10.1007/978-3-032-23089-8_8

such as age, fat content and tissue density, which must be considered when designing implants that are interacting mechanically with the breast [6]. Under compression, breast tissue shows anisotropic behavior, highlighting the importance of implant design that can distribute stress evenly and minimize local concentrations [7]. The development of a mechanically decoupled implant, consisting of an external load-bearing structure addresses mechanical requirements of the implant [8]. The external structure has to be designed in such way to act as a protective barrier, absorbing and distributing forces to safeguard the external structure, while the internal scaffold provides a favorable microenvironment for tissue regeneration and adipogenesis [9, 10]. The inclusion of a helicoidal "window" pattern in the external geometry is aimed to enhance vascularization and to facilitate nutrient exchange towards the inner core supporting fat graft survival and integration [11]. In terms of suitable materials to be used for 3D printing of such implant, there are several options to be considered, one of the suitable options for this particular case being the thermoplastic polyurethane (TPU) as this material is offering elasticity, resilience, and fatigue resistance, enabling the external structure to deform under load while returning to its original shape, mimicking the mechanical properties of natural breast tissue [12]. This material is suitable in the combination with the internal scaffold which is typically composed of bioresorbable polymers to provide structural support, biocompatibility, and tunable mechanical properties to promote adipose tissue growth [13]. The interplay between the external structure of the breast implant and the inner core of the scaffold is critical in terms of the elasticity in particular, as a low elastic modulus supports cell proliferation while maintaining structural mechanical resistance [14]. The architectural design of the implant including the number, diameter and arrangement of supporting arcs are influencing directly the load absorption and stress distribution in case of a breast implant [15]. Optimizing of these geometric parameters allows a balance between mechanical protection and tissue integration, supporting the development of patient-specific AM breast implants that meet long-term biomechanical requirements [16]. The paper aims to present several structural design variants of the external of the external structure of breast implant that were made by TPU 85A material by Fused Deposition Modeling Technology, structures that were mechanically tested at the compression later on for validating their mechanical behavior (in comparison with the results reached by finite element analysis) to have one appreciation on the reliability of Fused Deposition Modeling technology, the reached results being used in continuing for supplementary tests that are aimed to be realized in this domain in the future, related to mechanical, but also biological behavior of this implant (in particular of the inner core) for drugs administration.

2 Steps for Designing and Manufacturing Process of the Implant

The designing and manufacturing process of the proposed implant followed a structured workflow, as illustrated in Table 1.

As one may notice in Table 1, there were 7 steps that have been considered in this research concerning the breast implants, starting with MRI, designing and meshing of the models using 3D Slicer and Solidworks programs, followed by finite element analyses that were necessary to be done using SolidWorks simulation in order to determine the

Table. 1. Flowchart of the designing, manufacturing and testing of the breast implants

1. MRI scan/DICOM images →
2. Patient's breast 3D model (3D Slicer) →
3. SOLIDWORKS meshing - → Final CAD model of patient's breast →
4. Finite Element simulations to estimate the mechanical behavior at the compression →
5. Processing of the models for FDM printing (generating the STL and parameters)
6. FDM manufacturing
7. Mechanical testing at the compression for final validation

mechanical behavior at the compression, processing of the models for 3D printing and continuing with the manufacturing stage of the implants by Fused Deposition Modeling as well as mechanical testing at the compression that has been perfumed in the end, all these steps being presented in detail in continuing in the paper. As it has been mentioned, the process began with obtaining an MRI scan of a patient randomly and anonymously selected from cancerimagingarchive.net, which served as the initial dataset for implant design (see Fig. 1) [17]. The MRI data were exported in continuing into 3D Slicer software to reconstruct a three-dimensional model by assembling all sectional images (see Fig. 2), the resulted model after these operations being shown in Fig. 3.

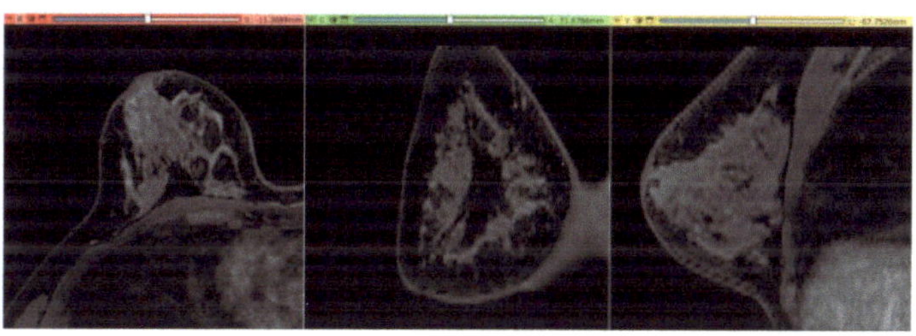

Fig. 1. DICOM images

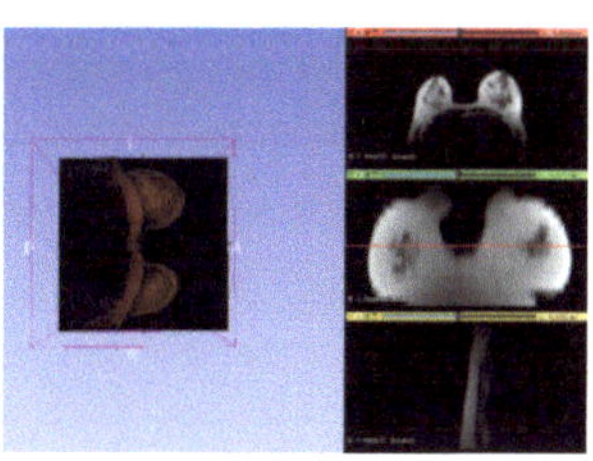

Fig. 2. Breast scan exported to 3D Slicer

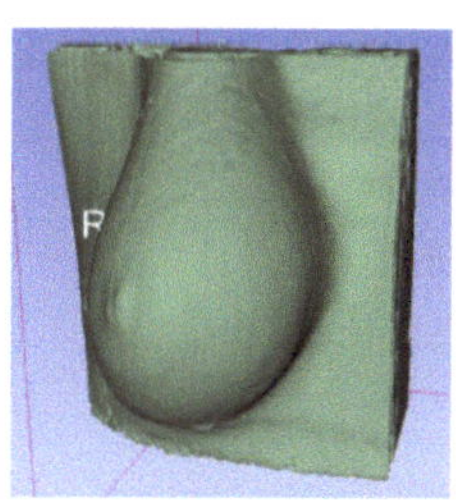

Fig. 3. 3D model generated from a specific MRI scan

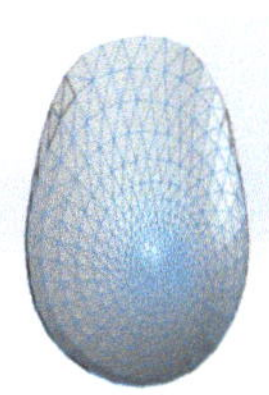

Fig. 4. Surface mesh of the 3D model

Further on in order to define the implant geometry, the reconstructed model was exported to SolidWorks, where a surface mesh was generated to serve as a reference for further design operations (see Fig. 4). This meshed surface provided the geometric foundation for developing the patient-specific implant. From the mechanical perspective, breast tissue exhibits elastic, compressible and viscoelastic properties, allowing it to deform under load and recover its original shape. These properties contribute to the uniform distribution of mechanical stress and enhance resilience. Fatigue resistance varies among individuals, depends on factors such as age, tissue density, lifestyle and medical conditions. In a simplified model, the elastic tissue can be represented as a spring supporting a mass equivalent to the breast weight.

3 Design of the External Structure of the Implant

The external structure of the implant was designed in continuing to protect the internal scaffold by attenuating mechanical loads, functioning similarly to a damping system. By reducing the impact transmitted to the core, the outer layer supports the conditions required for cellular growth. A helicoidally window pattern was adopted to enhance interaction between the internal scaffold and the vascularized environment. To minimize stress on the surrounding tissue, reducing implant weight was a priority. Therefore, the external frame was optimized to use as little material as possible while maintaining adequate structural protection. Instead of a full supporting platform, two semicircular "ears" were implemented to secure the internal core and facilitate assembly. The geometry consisted of a circular boundary with two semicircular clips, forming the base for attaching the arcs and the helicoidally elements, constrained to a hemispherical boundary surface with a diameter of approximately 80 mm, derived directly from the patient-specific mesh. Three design variants were developed using SolidWorks CAD program. While the general geometry remained constant, the number and diameter of the supporting arcs were modified to evaluate how these parameters influence compressive load absorption. Across the three models, the number of arc supports increased by roughly 90% from one version to the next, while the arc diameter was reduced accordingly. The specific design parameters are summarized in Table 2.

Table 2. Parameters of each model of the external structure

	Number of arcs	Arc diameter [mm]
Variant #1	4	5.6
Variant #2	7	5
Variant #3	14	3.2

The first structure design variant (see Fig. 5a) included four supporting arcs with a diameter of 5.6 mm, distributed equally at 45°, forming a cross-like arrangement when viewed from above. A helicoidally spiral starting from the center of the circular platform at 270°, with a 5.6 mm diameter and 10 revolutions with a 5 mm pitch have been realized, but due to the projection geometry only six revolutions have been materialized on the surface in this variant. The height of the circular platform was 4 mm. The ears of the platform had an 8 mm radius and an extension of 4 mm, summing up to a total 12 mm length from the tangent of the circular platform and a 2 mm height, to place the scaffold at the proper level inside the external structure.

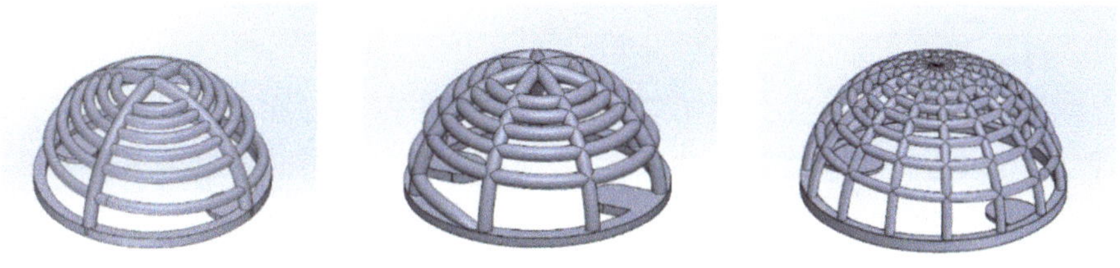

a. b. c.

Fig. 5. Geometrical views of the first (a), second (b) and third (c) variants

The second design variant for the external structure (see Fig. 5b.) had an increased number of arcs with a smaller diameter: seven arcs of 5 mm, equally distributed, with the first arc starting from 270°. Similarly, only 6 revolutions of the helicoidally spiral have been materialized on the boundary semi sphere. The rest of the parameters remained the same. For the third model the structural design shown in Fig. 5c variant was decided to be with fourteen arcs, each with a diameter of 3.4 mm. In this situation, out of ten revolutions projected, nine of them have been materialized, due to the smaller dimension of the arcs' diameter. The core model corresponding to the external structure is shown in Fig. 6. Initially, a solid hemispherical scaffold with a helicoidally channel was designed (see Fig. 7) being subsequently exported to Autodesk Fusion to generate a volumetric lattice structure. The lattice featured an "X"-shaped cell geometry with 3 mm cell size, were uniformly distributed throughout the volume.

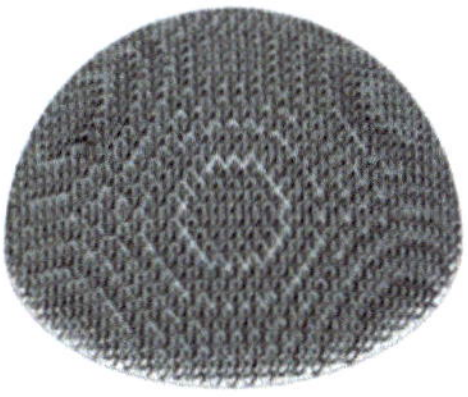

Fig. 6. Core scaffold structure

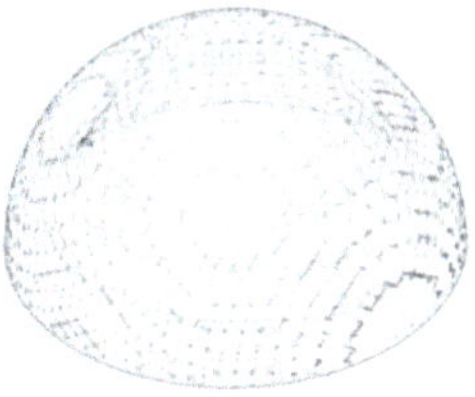

Fig. 7. Core scaffold with visible channel structure

The three-dimensional core structure was designed to support the adhesion and integration of injected adipose tissue. This internal scaffold also functions as a channel system integrated within the implant, being intended to deliver localized therapeutic agents in a controlled manner, thereby reducing the risk of cancer recurrence with minimal invasiveness. The design additionally is aimed to allow antibacterial coatings, antibiotics, local immunotherapy or oncolytic virus loading, particularly beneficial for post-lumpectomy cases. Finally, three complete assemblies were created (see Fig. 8a, b and c) to verify the spatial alignment and compatibility between the external structure and the internal scaffold.

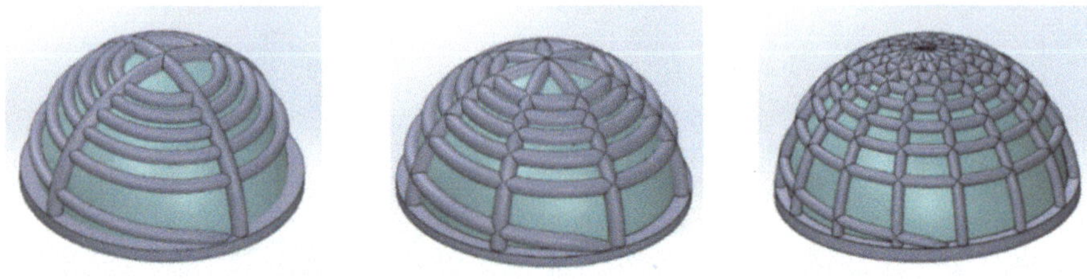

Fig. 8. Mechanically coupled implant with the first (a), second (b) and third (c) structure

4 Finite Element Analysis of the External Structures

A series of finite element analyses were conducted for each external structure of the implant model using SolidWorks simulation program in order to predict their behavior under compressive loading. In Table 3 are presented the material characteristics that were introduced into the system of TPU 85A material and the platen made out of steel AISI 1018 material that translates the force over the implant. TPU 85A and AISI 1018 material characteristics were taken from the technical data sheet of the producers of the materials [18, 19].

A circular platen (100 mm diameter, 5 mm thickness) was designed in SolidWorks CAD program to simulate the contact between a flat, rigid object and the implant, replicating the conditions of the mechanical tests. For each of the three external structures, assemblies were created with geometric constraints ensuring concentricity, parallelism and tangency between the platen and the highest surface point of the model. A static study was done in SolidWorks Simulation for each assembly. Boundary conditions included a fixed fixture on the bottom surface of the model so as to be in contact with the horizontal surface of the testing equipment and a second fixture was applied to the circular surrounding of the platen to ensure that it executes only a translation on Z axis. Contact definitions consisted of local interactions between the platen and the upper arcs of the model and global interactions treating each component as a separate body during meshing. A compressive load of 30 N was applied on the top surface of the platen, representing typical forces experienced during daily activities rather than total compression or structural failure [20] (see Fig. 9). Finally, a high-quality solid mesh with 16 Jacobian points was generated (see Fig. 10) to ensure accuracy and the simulations were run for all three models.

Following the setup of fixtures, compressive load, interactions, and meshing parameters, the analysis obtained results for total displacement, strain and stress as shown in

Table 3. Characteristics of each component

Implant #1		
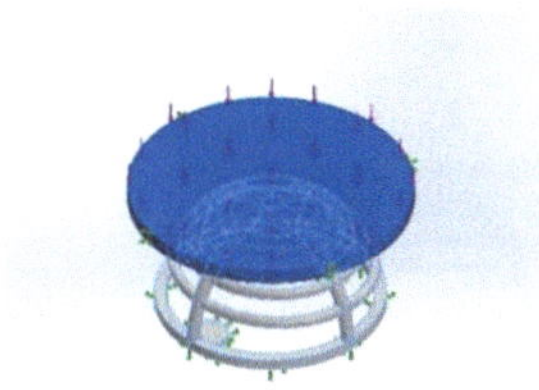	Name:	**TPU 85A**
	Model type:	**Linear Elastic Isotropic**
	Default failure criterion:	**Max von Mises Stress**
	Yield strength:	**4 MPa**
	Tensile strength:	**24 MPa**
	Elastic modulus:	**13 MPa**
	Poisson's ratio:	**0.4**
	Mass density:	**1.082 g/cm^3**
Platen		
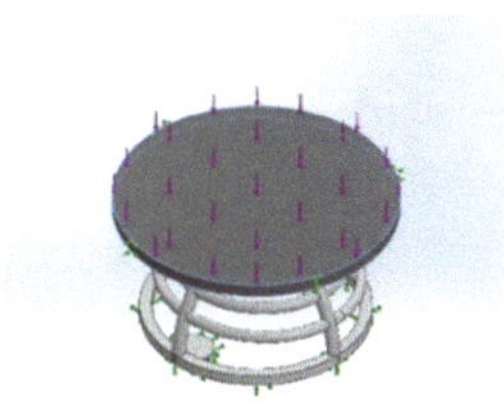	Name:	**Steel AISI 1018**
	Model type:	**Linear Elastic Isotropic**
	Default failure criterion:	**Max von Mises Stress**
	Yield strength:	**370 MPa**
	Tensile strength:	**440 MPa**
	Elastic modulus:	**205 GPa**
	Poisson's ratio:	**0.290**
	Mass density:	**7.87 g/cm^3**

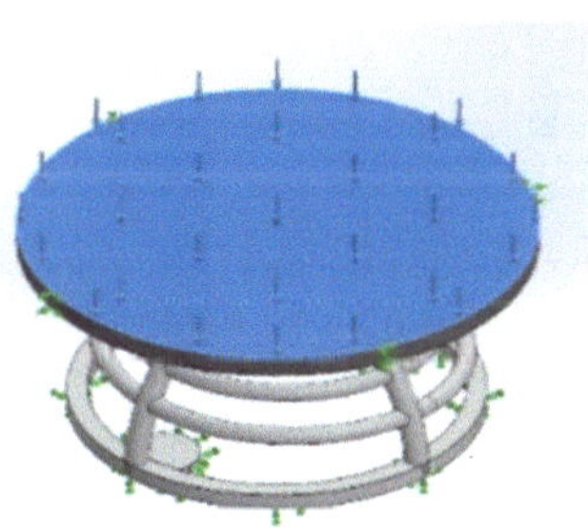

Fig. 9. Compressive load applied on the top surface of the platen

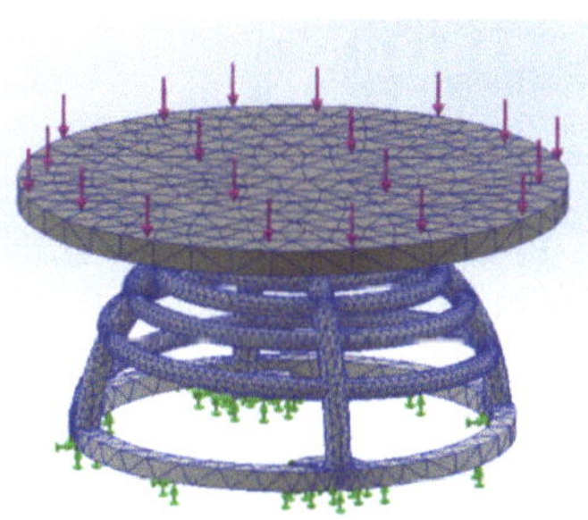

Fig. 10. Generated mesh

Fig. 11. As one may see in Fig. 11a, in case of first model variant, the total displacement was uniform, with a maximum value of 7.6 mm located at the top of the structure, at the crossing of the four arcs, and gradually decreasing toward the last helical revolution. The strain distribution (see Fig. 11b) indicated higher values in the regions joining the spiral and the arcs, ranging from 2.6% to 6.2%, with a maximum strain of 8.9% at the top arc intersection. The von Mises stress distribution shown in Fig. 11c followed a similar pattern, with the most affected areas corresponding to the high-strain regions. The maximum value of the stress obtained was 2.991 MPa in this case.

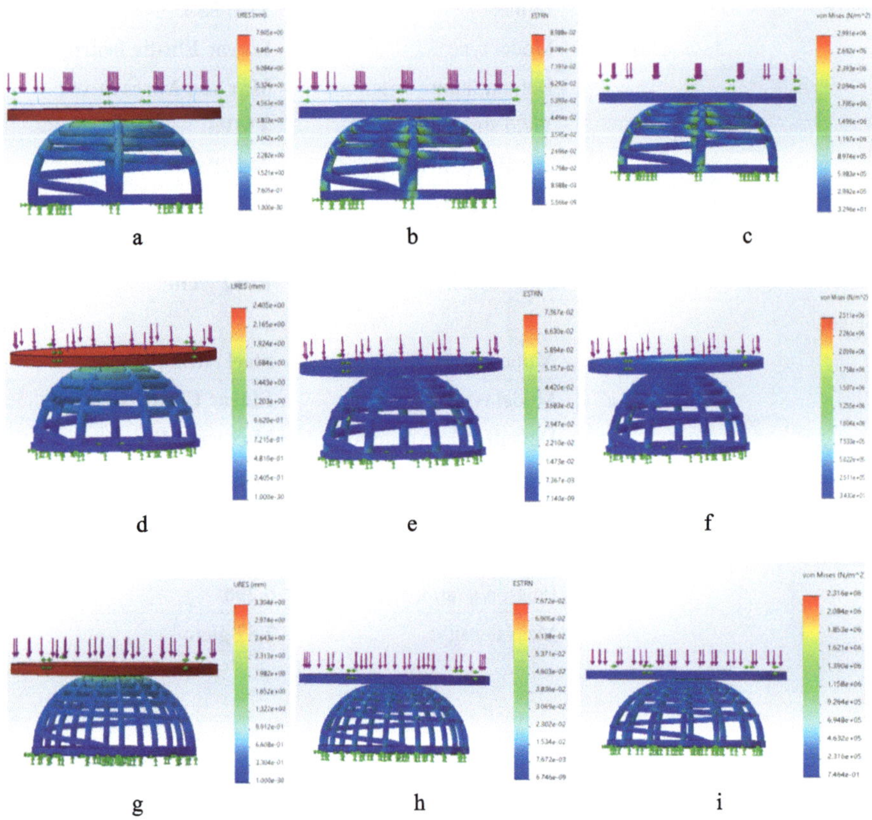

Fig. 11. Results of the finite element analysis concerning total displacement, strain and von Mises stress – (a-c) for the first variant, (d-f) for the second variant, (g-i) for the third variant

For the second variant, as one may notice in Fig. 11d the total displacement under the same 30 N compressive load showed a maximum value of 2.4 mm at the upper region lower than in the first model. The strain reached up to 7.36% as one may see in Fig. 11e, being mainly concentrated on the joints and the base of the arcs having a value of 7.36%. The maximum von Mises stress, identified in case of variant as shown in Fig. 11f was in the same areas as in case of variant 1, reaching out 2.511 MPa. In the case of the third model variant, the maximum total displacement under 30 N load was 3.3 mm a shown in Fig. 11g, being observed at the top center where the arcs intersecting and along the first three helical revolutions. The maximum strain reached 7.67% at the focal joints (see Fig. 11h), while the maximum von Mises stress obtained was 2.316 MPa as one may see in Fig. 11i. For the external structure to effectively protect the core scaffold from loads encountered during daily activities, the results must demonstrate that the structure can absorb stress efficiently, exhibit low displacement, and recover elastically without signs of permanent deformation. The stress–strain relationship obtained from the simulations is illustrated in Fig. 12. Based on these criteria, variant #2 achieved the most favorable outcome, showing a maximum stress of 2.511 MPa and a minimal total displacement of 2.4 mm. This configuration proved to be optimal for sustaining the 30 N compressive loads without significant distortion of the arcs or the helicoidally spiral. Finally, the implant is aimed to maintain adequate and resistant to external forces while avoiding excessive stiffness to mimic the natural mechanical properties of breast tissue.

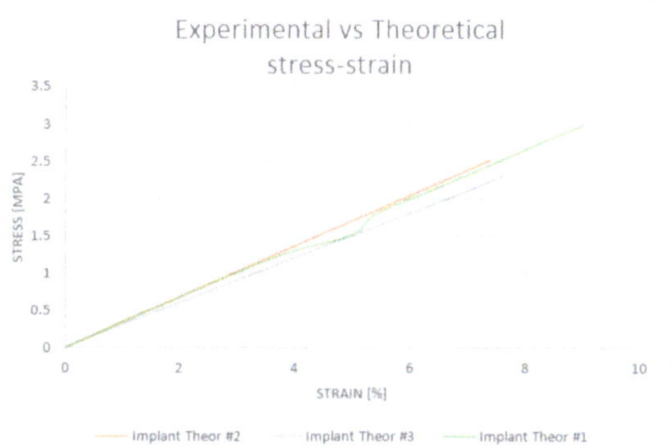

Fig. 12. Graphical representation of the stress-strain curve of the three implants

5 Manufacturing of the Breast Medical Implant by Fused Deposition Modeling

The implants were further on realized in the 3D Printing Laboratory at the Department of Manufacturing Engineering (Technical University of Cluj-Napoca, Romania). The models were printed with a Leapfrog Creatr HS dual-nozzle 3D printer (see Fig. 13). The filament used for the exterior structure was medical grade UltraFuse TPU 85A 750 g. To optimize print quality, the infill density was decreased from 25% to 20%, to compensate for slower deposition velocity and not lower so that the porosity of the structure will not be compromised. Due to the complex geometry, support structures were required to sustain the spiral and arcs during fabrication. These were designed with a pyramidal geometry to ensure stability while minimizing material usage and post-processing effort. During post-processing of the 3D printed structures, time efficiency proved to be a significant challenge. The elastic and fracture resistant nature of TPU combined with the fragility of certain regions, required frequent alternation between two types of cutters and a specialized scissor. This increased processing time and demanded significant physical force to maintain constant restraint and torque with the clamp during cutting. Overall, the post-processing of all three implants required approximately three hours, with an average of one hour per model. The final variants of all three external structure of breast implants after post-processing are shown in Fig. 14.

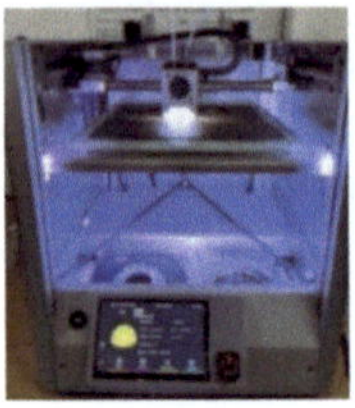

Fig. 13. Leapfrog Creatr HS printer

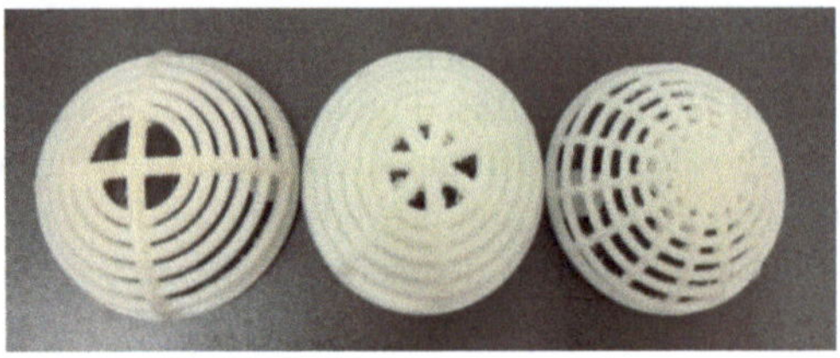

Fig. 14. The three printed implants after post-processing

Although all implants were successfully printed, several complications and deviations from the standard design were observed in their final printed structures. The first variant exhibited the most uniform and consistent geometry, followed by the second variant, which presented a few minor defects, and finally the third variant, which showed the highest porosity and most defective areas. Most of the gaps and shape irregularities were concentrated at the base of the implants, right where the formation of the arc began. Based on the pattern of irregularities it was concluded that smaller arc diameters tend to generate larger gaps and more printing errors in the structure of the implants.

6 Mechanical Testing of the Breast Medical Implants at Compression

A series of uniaxial compression tests were conducted on the 3D printed models to obtain experimental data and evaluate how the structures respond to external loads.

The tests were performed at the Mechanical Testing laboratory from the Faculty of the Automotive, Mechatronics and Mechanical Engineering (Technical University of Cluj-Napoca, Romania) using an Instron 3366 testing machine, equipped with two circular rigid platens, one fixed and one movable. This setup simulated the contact between a rigid object and the breast, allowing for controlled and repeatable testing conditions. Each printed implant was placed concentrically on the marked area of the fixed platen. To replicate the compressive forces acting on a breast implant, the movable platen was lowered at a constant displacement rate of 0.1 mm/s. Figure 15 illustrates the implants before and during the compression process.

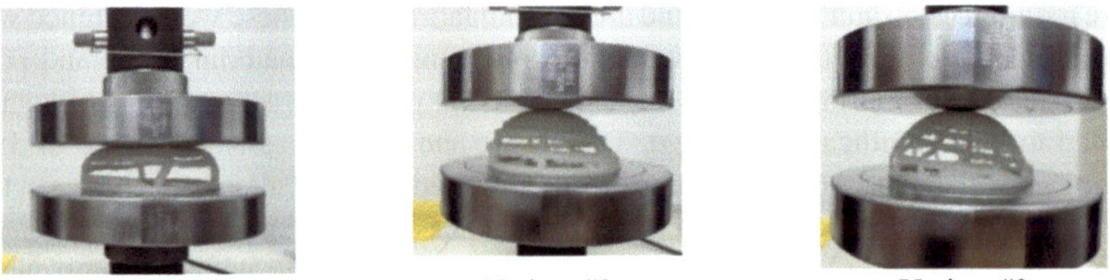

Variant #1 Variant #2 Variant #3

Fig. 15. Breast implants during compression mechanical testing

The purpose of these implants, which are the exterior structures of the implant, was to find the values of the characteristics that will absorb a great part of the stressing force while maintaining the natural mechanical properties of a breast. As one may notice in Fig. 16, the highest value registered for the maximum compressive load was found in the case of the second exterior structure model, represented in the graph with orange as Breast Implant (Specimen #2) at 32 N with a corresponding compressive extension of 15 mm. The compressive load-extension curve for the second structure of breast implant appeared to be the most uniform when ascending to the maximum compressive load value, while maintaining a proportional displacement.

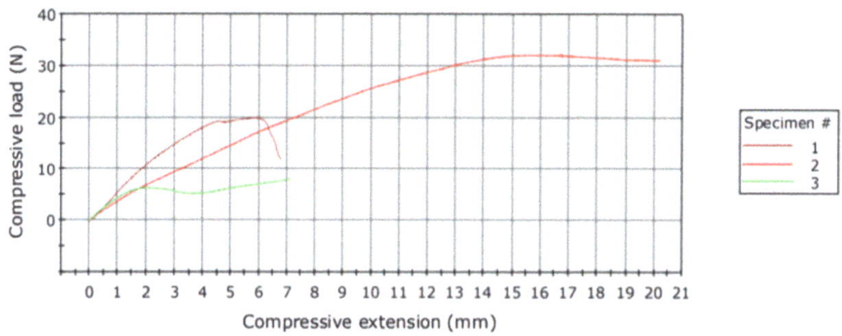

Fig. 16. Graphical representation of the compressive load-extension curve

The first variant testing result in Fig. 16 is marked on the graph with a purple line, where the maximum compressive load registered almost reached 20 N with a corresponding compressive extension of 5.9 mm. Although the displacement was lower, the maximum load can absorb is just 20 N, significantly smaller than the second variant of the implant. Ultimately, as shown in Fig. 16, the lowest force absorption was noted in the case of the third variant, at a maximum compressive load of 8 N, with a corresponding compressive extension of 7 mm. The behavior of the third structure of the breast implant is visually represented with a green curve. The slope of its load extension curve was higher than that of the second variant of the implant but lower than the first variant, reflecting its reduced structural strength. After performing the compression tests, all three implants returned to their initial form, TPU 85A being flexible and resistant to shear stress, no visible tears or damages appeared due to the compressive load. Out of all implants, the most unfavorable behavior was presented by Variant #3, which had an 8 N load absorption, in contrast with Variant #2, which reached the best mechanical characteristics, having the capacity to absorb a 32 N compression load.

7 Conclusions

The proposed implant developed in this research was designed as a mechanically decoupled system composed of an external load-bearing structure and an internal regenerative scaffold, addressing biomechanical requirements for long-term breast tissue regeneration and the prevention of malignant cell recurrence. Using Fused Deposition Modeling

(FDM) and TPU 85A medical-grade material, the design aimed to ensure mechanical characteristics that are specific to the external structure of breast type implant. The external structure, featuring a circular, multi-arched geometry has been designed in this way in order to determine which of the designed variants leads to the best load absorption. Three structural variants of the external shell were produced to assess the influence of geometry on stiffness and deformation behavior under a 30 N compressive load. Finite Element Analysis indicated that the second variant exhibited the lowest displacement (2.4 mm) and the most favorable mechanical response to the loading stresses. Although experimental tests revealed deviations from simulation results due to printing defects, results reached on the mechanical tests that have been made at compression have led to the same conclusion that the second variant is the one that is providing superior mechanical performance as compared with the other variants that have been considered in this research. The highest stress concentration areas were observed at the arc–spiral junctions, suggesting that smaller-diameter, higher-count arc configurations enhances load distribution in these particular areas.

Acknowledgments. This research was supported by the ERASMUS+ Partnerships for cooperation and exchanges of practices (KA220) -"Biomedical Innovations through Digital Transformation of Additive Technologies and Knowledge Exchange - BIOMEDIX" -Project No. 2024-1-LV01-KA220-HED-000255929.

References

1. Babu RD, Devaprakasam D (2019) A review on additive manufacturing techniques in medical applications. Int J Adv Sci Eng 5(3):988–997
2. Medellín-Castillo HI, Zaragoza-Siqueiros J (2019) Design and manufacturing strategies for fused deposition modelling in additive manufacturing: a review. Chin J Mech Eng 32:53
3. Teixeira AM, Martins P (2023) A review of bioengineering techniques applied to breast tissue: mechanical properties, tissue engineering and finite element analysis. Front Bioeng Biotechnol 11:1161815
4. Kiseleva V et al (2025) Three-dimensional disassemblable scaffolds for breast reconstruction. Polymers 17(15):2036
5. Muñoz Avendaño ALE (2023) Literature review on the different types of breast implants: advantages and disadvantages. Int. J Medical Sci Clin Res Stud 03(05):990–994
6. Perera D et al (2024) The distribution of breast density in women aged 18 years and older. Breast Cancer Res Treat 205:521–531
7. Serwan E, Matthews D, Davies J, Chau M (2020) Mammographic compression practices of force- and pressure-standardisation protocol: a scoping review. J Med Radiat Sci 67:233–242
8. Tonekaboni S, Friedman SF, Zhang X, Maddah M, Uhler C (2025) A representation fusion framework for decoupling diagnostic information in multimodal learning. Digital Med 8:765
9. Lee S et al (2025) A computational framework for investigating the mechanical stresses on breast implants under dynamic loading conditions. Ann Biomed Eng 53:3096–3108
10. Chae MP, Hunter-Smith DJ, Murphy SV, Findlay MW (2017) 3D bioprinting adipose tissue for breast reconstruction. In: Thomas DJ, Jessop ZM, Whitaker IS (eds) 3D bioprinting for reconstructive surgery: techniques and applications. Academic Press, pp 305–353
11. Zibold F et al (2009) Surface dose in the treatment of breast cancer with helical tomotherapy. Strahlenther Onkol 185:574–581

12. Burke A, Hasirci N (2004) Polyurethanes in biomedical applications. In: Hasirci N, Hasirci V (eds) Biomaterials: advances in experimental medicine and biology, vol 553. Springer, Boston, MA, pp 83–101
13. Auque A, Bodin F (2025) Comparative study between breast implants and adipose tissue autograft in primary aesthetic breast augmentation. Aesth Plast Surg 49:6290–6302
14. Samani A, Zubovits J, Plewes D (2007) Elastic moduli of normal and pathological human breast tissues: an inversion-technique-based investigation of 169 samples. Phys Med Biol 52(6):1565–1586
15. Garbey M, Thanoon D, Salmon RS, Bass B (2011) Multi-scale modeling and computational surgery: application to breast conservative therapy. J Serbian Soc Comput Mech 5(2):81–89
16. Harding A, Pramanik A, Basak AK, Prakash C, Shankar S (2023) Application of additive manufacturing in the biomedical field- a review, annals of 3D. Print Med 10:100110
17. The Cancer Imaging Archive. https://www.cancerimagingarchive.net. Last accessed 7 Nov 2025
18. AISI 1018 Mild/Low Carbon Steel material characteristics. https://esmusa.elwd.com/wp-content/uploads/2013/10/1018.pdf. Last accessed 7 Nov 2025
19. Ultrafuse TPU 85A TDS EN v2.0 material characteristics. https://www.printam3d.ro/media/productattachment/0/1669/UltrafuseTPU85ATDSENv20.pdf. Last accessed 7 Nov 2025
20. Typical forces experienced in case of breast implants. https://www.tainstruments.com/pdf/literature/EF001.pdf. Last accessed 7 Nov 2025

Design and Strength Analysis of a Mechanical Wrist Orthosis for Tremor Suppression

Bora Kutlu(✉) and Michał Rychlik

Poznan University of Technology, Institute of Applied Mechanics, Poznan, Poland
bora.kutlu@doctorate.put.poznan.pl

Abstract. Tremor disorders can severely limit fine motor control and daily independence. While medications and physical therapy may reduce symptoms, they often involve side effects, adherence challenges, and inconsistent outcomes, especially after stroke. Orthotic devices offer immediate, non-drug support; active systems provide adaptive assistance but tend to be heavy, expensive, and maintenance intensive, whereas passive devices are simpler and more reliable yet must balance stabilization with comfort, adjustability, and long-term wearability. This study presents a purely mechanical, low-profile, modular wrist orthosis designed for tremor and dystonia management, customized from patient-specific 3D anatomy, developed through CAD, and produced using additive and incremental manufacturing methods. Design evaluation includes finite element analyses and prototype testing focused on fit, usability, and preliminary functional performance. The work emphasizes reliability, ease of use, and user autonomy without reliance on power or electronics, and outlines a pathway for refinement, clinical testing, and integration into personalized motor-rehabilitation strategies.

Keywords: tremor · wrist orthosis · passive mechanical stabilization · additive manufacturing · finite element analysis · patient-specific design

1 Introduction and Background

1.1 Purpose and Context

Wrist tremor and post–stroke dystonia degrade fine motor control, reduce independence, and limit performance in daily activities such as eating, writing, and personal care. Orthotic solutions can mitigate these effects by stabilizing the joint, yet clinical adoption depends on comfort, ease of use, durability, and the ability to preserve voluntary motion when stabilization is not needed. This study addresses these requirements by developing a compact, purely mechanical wrist orthosis that can be selectively engaged to suppress tremor while remaining unobtrusive in daily wear.

In contrast to active and semi-active tremor suppression systems that rely on sensors, actuators, and control electronics, this study investigates a purely mechanical, patient-specific solution enabled by digital anatomical modelling and additive manufacturing. By leveraging subject-specific geometry and material tuning, the proposed approach

F. Górski et al. (Eds.): MANUFACTURING 2026, LNME, pp. 100–114, 2026.
https://doi.org/10.1007/978-3-032-23089-8_9

aims to achieve effective tremor attenuation while maintaining autonomy, robustness, and ease of use. This positions the presented orthosis as a lightweight and clinically viable alternative for users who require reliable tremor mitigation without external power supply or complex control architectures.

1.2 Background and Gaps

Orthoses can be grouped as active, semi-active, or passive systems. Active devices employ powered actuators with feedback control to reject tremor, which increases mass, complexity, and maintenance burden [1]. Semi-active designs modulate resistance with tunable elements such as magnetorheological dampers, offering adaptability at lower power cost. Passive solutions rely on mechanical means such as frictional interfaces, viscoelastic layers, or tuned masses to dissipate energy and are attractive for their simplicity and silent operation [2, 3].

Despite progress, three gaps persist. First, many commercial braces are not patient specific, which leads to pressure concentrations and poor long-term tolerance. Second, devices that rely on strap tension or hinge friction seldom provide discrete, repeatable end-stops with a crisp feel at engagement. Third, additive manufacturing is under-utilized for creating lightweight, ventilated, and modular architectures that support part-level replacement and upgrades. These gaps motivate a design that combines personalized shells with a compact mechanical locking mechanism located at a defined interface, so stabilization is precise when required and the joint remains free otherwise.

1.3 Biomechanical Anchor and Scope

Design targets were anchored to wrist biomechanics typical of daily functional tasks and tremor suppression needs. Range-of-motion limits were respected to keep neutral comfort, and loading for verification used combined flexion–extension (WFE) and abduction–adduction (WAA) moments representative of wrist-level disturbances observed in practice. In the computational campaign, load cases employed sequential ramps of $\pm 7.0 \times 10^3$ N·mm for WFE and $\pm 3.0 \times 10^3$ N·mm for WAA, together with localized interface pressures up to 0.08 MPa for comfort screening. The analysis compared two locking-set materials—SLA resin and binder-jetted 316 L stainless steel—while keeping the patient-specific shells in FDM PLA. Prototype-level checks covered mass, comfort, donning and doffing, and qualitative stabilization during common tasks.

1.4 Scope of the Study

The scope of this study comprises:

- patient-specific geometric modelling and a modular, low-profile orthosis architecture tailored to tremor suppression;
- selection and pairing of materials and manufacturing processes for the polymer shells and mechanical locking components;
- non-linear finite element simulations incorporating frictional contact to evaluate deformation, stress distribution, contact pressure, and safety factors under physiological moment loading;

- benchtop validation and on-patient observations to assess donning feasibility, comfort, and functional usability.

The study places particular emphasis on a mixed-material design strategy, combining lightweight polymer shells for ergonomics with metal locking elements for precision, stability, and long-term durability.

1.5 Objectives and Hypotheses

Objective. To design, fabricate, and evaluate a modular, low-profile wrist orthosis that suppresses tremor using a purely mechanical locking mechanism without electronics or external power.

Hypotheses

1. A patient-specific shell combined with a discrete locking mechanism will limit peak total deformation to about 0.3 mm under representative wrist moments, while keeping shell stresses below PLA yield.
2. Replacing an SLA resin locking set with 316 L stainless steel will increase local stiffness, concentrate contact pressure in a smaller footprint, and raise the minimum safety factor to ≥ 1.85 across the critical step, without pushing total worn mass beyond $\sim 105 \pm 3$ g.
3. The modular architecture will preserve natural wrist motion when unlocked and provide a repeatable, precise end stop when locked, improving subjective stability during representative daily tasks.

2 Literature Review

The development of a purely mechanical wrist orthosis for tremor stabilization requires integration of clinical tremor characteristics, upper-limb biomechanics, and orthotic engineering. While prior studies report significant advances, limitations persist in multi-axis stabilization, wearability, and patient-specific adaptability. This section summarizes the clinical background, biomechanical considerations, and existing orthotic approaches motivating the present work.

2.1 Clinical and Biomechanical Background

Tremor disorders are involuntary rhythmic oscillations that impair fine motor control, most commonly associated with Essential Tremor (ET), Parkinsonian tremor, and post-stroke tremor. ET typically occurs during voluntary motion and may progress beyond the upper limb, whereas Parkinsonian tremor predominantly appears at rest and exhibits lower frequency and asymmetry [4–7]. Post-stroke tremor affects approximately 1–4% of patients and often presents mixed activation modes depending on lesion location [8–10]. These motor impairments frequently coexist with depression and anxiety, further degrading quality of life [11, 12].

From a biomechanical perspective, tremor primarily manifests in wrist and forearm motion. The upper limb exhibits seven principal degrees of freedom (DOFs): shoulder flexion–extension, abduction–adduction, internal–external rotation, elbow flexion–extension, forearm pronation–supination (FPS), wrist flexion–extension (WFE), and wrist radial–ulnar deviation (WRUD) [5, 13, 14]. Kinetic tremors typically show the largest amplitudes in FPS and WFE.

A simplified dynamic model of a single-DOF joint is given by

$$J\theta^{\cdot\cdot} + \beta\theta^{\cdot} + \kappa\theta = T_m(r) + T_e, \quad (1)$$

where J is rotational inertia, β viscous damping, and κ joint stiffness [15, 16]. This formulation emphasizes resonance effects and the role of mechanical constraints in tremor attenuation [17, 18].

2.2 Existing Orthotic Technologies

Orthoses for tremor suppression are generally categorized as active, semi-active, or passive. Active systems employ powered actuators with closed-loop control [1, 19], while semi-active designs use adjustable damping elements such as magnetorheological or pneumatic components [20, 21]. Passive orthoses rely solely on mechanical mechanisms including friction, viscoelastic damping, or tuned-mass absorbers [2, 3, 22, 23].

Although active and semi-active devices provide precise control, they are penalized by increased mass, cost, energy demand, and maintenance requirements [24, 25]. Passive systems offer superior robustness and simplicity but are typically limited to single-DOF stabilization and lack ergonomic adaptability [26]. As summarized in Table 1, compact, mechanical-only multi-axis orthoses suitable for prolonged daily use remain largely absent, underscoring the need for lightweight, patient-specific solutions.

Table 1. Summary of orthotic systems, actuation type, and DOF coverage [27]

Orthosis / Group	Control Type	DOF Coverage
Voluntary-Driven Orthosis [28]	Active	1/1 (EFE)
EMG Exoskeleton [29, 30]	Active	1/4 (EFE)
WOTAS [1, 31]	Active	3/4 (no WD)
ADL Exoskeleton [24]	Active	2/3 (WFE, FPS)
MR Damper Orthosis [21]	Semi-active	4/4
Pneumatic Hand Cuff [32]	Semi-active	2/2 (WFE, WD)
DVB Orthosis [33]	Semi-active	2/2 (WFE, WD)
Viscous Beam [2]	Passive	1/2 (WFE)
Air Dashpot Orthosis [3]	Passive	3/4 (no FPS)
Vib-Bracelet [22, 23]	Passive	1/1 (FPS)

2.3 Materials and Manufacturing Strategies

Material selection is critical for balancing stiffness, mass, and comfort. Thermoplastics such as PLA and PET-G provide structural rigidity, while TPU enables localized compliance in pressure-sensitive regions [34]. SLA resins offer high precision for locking components, and binder-jetted 316 L stainless steel enables durable metallic interfaces where higher strength is required [35, 36]. Additive manufacturing supports perforated and lattice geometries that reduce mass and improve breathability, complemented by soft liners and textiles that distribute pressure and regulate moisture [37, 38].

2.4 Identified Gaps and Design Motivation

Despite extensive research, key limitations persist: the lack of fully mechanical multiaxis tremor suppression, limited ergonomic adaptability across users, and underutilization of additive manufacturing for patient-specific customization. Active systems compromise simplicity and autonomy, while passive solutions rarely provide personalization or selective stabilization [26, 39]. These gaps motivate the development of a lightweight, modular, power-free orthosis capable of delivering selective mechanical tremor stabilization.

3 Methodology

This section outlines the end-to-end development of a compact, purely mechanical wrist orthosis, encompassing anatomical acquisition, CAD modelling, material selection, numerical verification, and prototype evaluation. The workflow followed a structured sequence: *requirements → 3D scanning → CAD design → finite element analysis → additive manufacturing and testing*. Emphasis was placed on manufacturability, usability, and reproducibility to support clinical translation.

3.1 Design Concept and Functional Requirements

The objective was to develop a low-profile, purely mechanical wrist orthosis that selectively stabilizes tremor while preserving voluntary motion, long-term comfort, and manufacturability. Functional requirements were derived from biomechanical literature, patient feedback, and prior orthotic research. Tremor suppression was achieved through a manual locking mechanism acting at the wrist flexion–extension (WFE) and abduction–adduction (WAA) interfaces. A patient-specific fit was ensured using high resolution 3D scanning with mirrored anatomical reconstruction. To minimize mass and improve ventilation, the shell employed a perforated architecture with wall thicknesses of 2–4 mm. Usability and serviceability were supported through a modular component layout with magnetic alignment aids, while mechanical reliability was addressed through a mixed-material strategy and verified using non-linear finite element analysis.

3.2 Anatomical Acquisition and CAD Architecture

Anatomical geometry was captured using an iReal M3 infrared scanner in neutral wrist posture. Due to mild dystonia, the contralateral limb was scanned and digitally mirrored. Mesh processing included automated hole filling, smoothing, and curvature preserving reconstruction.

Patient-specific CAD modelling (Autodesk Fusion 360) employed longitudinal slicing, spline-based cross-section reconstruction, and generation of a smooth inner shell. Modular locking components and an engagement rod enabled manual on/off tremor suppression. The resulting geometry directly informed both numerical analysis and additive fabrication.

3.3 Material Selection and Properties

Material–process pairing ensured adequate strength-to-weight ratio and manufacturbility.

A unified dataset was used for all simulations and prototypes (Table 2).

Table 2. Baseline material properties used in modelling

Property	PLA (FDM)	SLA Resin	316 L SS
Density (kg/mm^3)	1.24×10^{-6}	1.15×10^{-6}	8.00×10^{-6}
Young's modulus (MPa)	3300	2500	200000
Poisson's ratio	0.36	0.41	0.29
Yield strength (MPa)	45	35	219
Ultimate strength (MPa)	55	50	561

3.4 Finite Element Modelling and Boundary Conditions

Non-linear static analyses were performed in ANSYS Workbench 2024 with large deflection kinematics and contact. Two locking configurations (SLA resin and 316 L) were modeled with identical PLA shells.

Boundary Conditions. The distal forearm shell was fixed, while opposing wrist moments simulated tremor amplitudes based on clinical ranges [13, 18]:

$$M_{\mathrm{WFE}} = \pm(7.0 \pm 0.2) \times 103\ \mathrm{N \cdot mm},$$

$$M_{\mathrm{WAA}} = \pm(3.0 \pm 0.1) \times 103\ \mathrm{N \cdot mm}. \quad (2)$$

Contacts and Mesh. Lock interfaces were frictional ($\mu = 0.5$), shell–shell semi-bonded ($\mu = 0.2$), and rods no-separation. Lock components were meshed with hex-dominant elements (0.8 mm refinement) and the shell with tetrahedral elements (1.5 mm), achieving >0.85 average element quality.

Outputs included deformation fields, stress maps, strain energy, contact pressures, and safety factors.

3.5 Prototype Fabrication and Evaluation

Shells were FDM-printed in PLA, locks fabricated by SLA and binder-jetted 316 L for strength trials. Assembly used press-fit and adhesive bonding at lock interfaces.

Testing Protocol. A post-stroke participant performed daily-activity simulations under physiotherapist supervision:

- **Fit/comfort:** 2 h continuous wear; monitored pressure points and heat buildup.
- **Usability:** donning/doffing time, tactile feedback, and ease of manual locking.
- **Functional performance:** tremor suppression during eating, drinking, and handwriting tasks.

Measurement uncertainties were estimated at ± 0.1 mm (geometry) and $\pm 5\%$ (loads). Results of numerical and experimental tests are summarized in the following section.

4 Results

This section summarizes the principal outcomes of numerical and experimental evaluation of the proposed wrist orthosis. Results are grouped into numerical (finite element) analyses and experimental prototype validation to enable direct comparison between predicted and observed behaviour. All simulation material parameters are listed in Table 2 for clarity and reproducibility.

4.1 3D Model and Design Parameters

The analyzed assembly combined patient-specific PLA shells (forearm and hand) with a modular locking set comprising an engagement rod, receiver lock, base lock, and stabilizer. Cosmetic features and non-structural fillets were suppressed, while perforations and functional radii were retained to preserve representative stiffness. Local refinement at the locking interfaces and distal margins produced approximately 3.0×10^5 elements with characteristic sizes of 0.8–1.5 mm.

The forearm shell was fully constrained, and opposing sequential moments emulated combined wrist flexion–extension (WFE) and abduction–adduction (WAA) tremor motion: $\pm(7.0 \pm 0.2) \times 10^3$ N·mm (WFE) and $\pm$ $(3.0 \pm 0.1) \times 10^3$ N·mm (WAA). Contacts were frictional at the lock interfaces ($\mu = 0.5$) and between polymer shells ($\mu =$ 0.2). Material properties (Table 2) were applied consistently; 316 L was elastic–plastic with bilinear hardening, while PLA and SLA were linear-elastic.

4.2 Numerical Validation

Finite element simulations quantified deformation, stress, contact response, and safety margins for two locking-mechanism material variants (SLA resin and binder-jetted 316 L stainless steel) under combined WFE/WAA moments representative of tremor amplitudes reported in the literature [13, 18]. The results below compare deformation fields, yield margins, and rod–receiver interface pressures.

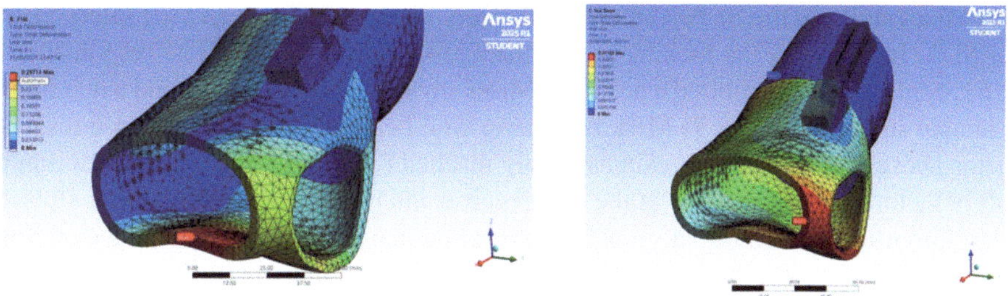

(a) 316L: total deformation (b) SLA: total deformation

Fig. 1. Visualization of peak total deformation fields under combined WFE/WAA loading

Global Deformation. Figure 1 shows that peak deformation localized near the distal housing in both material configurations. The 316 L locking mechanism limited total displacement to (0.30 ± 0.02) mm, while the SLA version reached (0.41 ± 0.03) mm. Directional components (X, Y, Z) followed the same pattern, with smaller and more confined deflection regions in the 316 L model, consistent with its higher elastic modulus (200 GPa vs. 2.5 GPa for SLA).

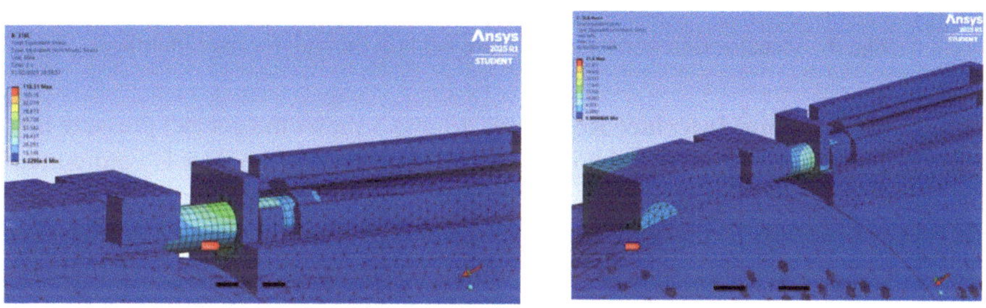

(a) 316L: von Mises stress (b) SLA: von Mises stress

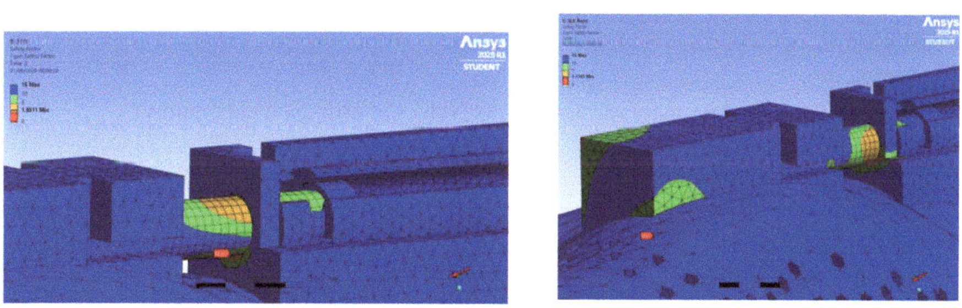

(c) 316L: safety factor (d) SLA: safety factor

Fig. 2. Visualization of stress and safety factor distributions for both material variants at the critical load step

Yield Margins and Control Region. Figure 2 presents the stress and safety factor distributions for both material variants: (a) von Mises stress in the 316 L assembly, (b)

von Mises stress in the SLA assembly, (c) safety factor for 316 L, and (d) safety factor for SLA. In all cases, the locking mechanism governed the global stress response. The 316 L configuration exhibited a peak von Mises stress of (118 ± 5) MPa and a maximum principal stress of (147 ± 7) MPa, remaining well below yield with a minimum safety factor above 1.85. The SLA resin assembly reached (31 ± 3) MPa, with the minimum safety factor approaching 1.1 at the rod–receiver interface. Although polymer stresses were lower, localized strain accumulation resulted in greater elastic compliance during load reversal, whereas the 316 L lock provided stiffer and more predictable mechanical control.

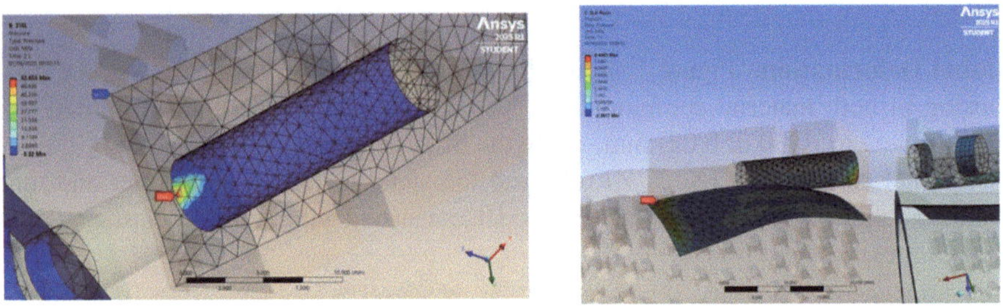

(a) 316L: contact pressure (b) SLA: contact pressure

Fig. 3. Visualization of contact pressure fields at the rod–receiver interface

Contact Pressure and Interface Response. Figure 3 shows the contact pressure fields at the rod–receiver interface for both material variants: (a) the 316 L configuration and (b) the SLA resin configuration. The material-dependent trend mirrors the stiffness differences observed in the global response. The 316 L assembly produced concentrated pressure zones exceeding (52 ± 3) MPa, indicating crisp seating and high wear resistance. The SLA variant distributed pressure more broadly, with local peaks near (8.4 ± 0.7) MPa, resulting in smoother engagement but reduced positional repeatability. Both configurations remained below the elastic indentation limits of their respective materials.

Table 3. Summary of FEA results (values ± estimated uncertainty)

Metric	316 L Assembly	SLA Assembly
Total deformation	0.30 ± 0.02 mm	0.41 ± 0.03 mm
Engagement rod deflection	0.038 ± 0.002 mm	0.35 ± 0.03 mm
Von Mises stress	118 ± 5 MPa	31 ± 3 MPa
Principal stress	147 ± 7 MPa	30 ± 2 MPa
Contact pressure	52 ± 3 MPa	8.4 ± 0.7 MPa
Min. safety factor	>1.85	1.1 ± 0.1
Shell stress (PLA)	<35 MPa	<35 MPa

Component-Level Summary. As summarized in Table 3, all stresses remained below material limits, validating both mixed-material configurations. The 316 L assembly demonstrated the highest stiffness, minimal deformation, and superior safety margins, confirming its suitability for long-term use and repeatable mechanical locking. In contrast, the SLA prototype retained adequate strength for short-term trials and rapid iteration but exhibited larger elastic offsets and lower fatigue potential.

4.3 Experimental Validation

Prototypes followed the same material pairing as simulation (FDM PLA shells with SLA locks, and 316 L locks for the metal validation). Functional tests were conducted with a post-stroke participant exhibiting mild tremor to evaluate comfort, alignment, and stabilization in daily activities. Although no quantitative tremor metrics were recorded, qualitative task performance, user-reported stability, and consistent observational outcomes provided a coherent basis for evaluating mechanical effectiveness.

Strength and Stability. The assembled orthosis withstood repeated drops from ~1 m and short-term ambient exposure without cracking or discolouration. Lock engagement remained stable over 50 manual cycles. In agreement with simulation, the SLA variant exhibited perceptible compliance at engagement, whereas 316 L produced a sharper end stop with minimal play.

Comfort and User Feedback. A ~3 h continuous wear test by the post-stroke participant confirmed acceptable comfort, with localized irritation indicating the need for moisture-managing liners. Unlocked mode preserved natural wrist motion, while locked mode enabled repeatable stabilization during eating and handwriting tasks. Locking precision was rated higher for the metal variant due to clearer tactile feedback. Occasional misalignment during rapid donning highlighted the need for passive alignment guides such as keyed rails or shallow tapers.

4.4 Long-Term Use and Durability Observations

Beyond short-term checks, the prototype was intermittently used for approximately six months by the same participant during daily activities to assess wear behaviour. The locking mechanism remained fully functional, with no observable reduction in engagement quality, loss of stiffness, structural damage, or increase in play. Manual locking and unlocking were repeated throughout use (conservatively several thousand cycles) without mechanical failure.

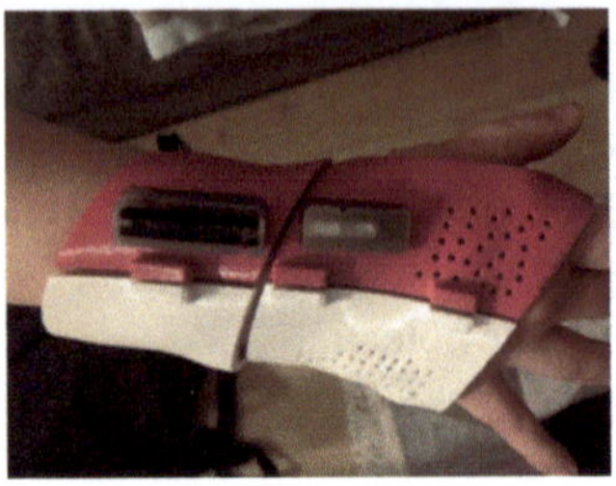

(a) Orthosis worn by the user in unlocked mode during dimensional evaluation.

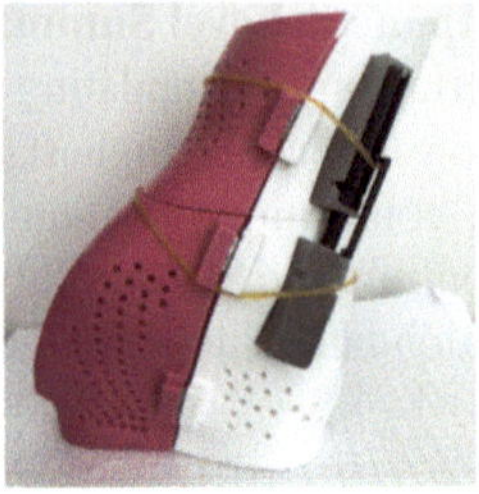

(b) Printed prototype with temporarily attached SLA locking mechanism.

Fig. 4. Final additively manufactured patient-specific wrist orthosis used in the experimental validation. The figure illustrates the modular architecture, mixed-material configuration, and the assembled prototype as tested by the user

Figure 4 shows the printed prototype used for validation. As shown in Fig. 4a, the orthosis could be worn in the unlocked state while preserving natural wrist motion, and the printed shells and modular interfaces remained intact during daily use. Figure 4b illustrates the modular architecture with temporarily installed SLA locks used to evaluate alignment and engagement prior to final integration, revealing donning-related alignment sensitivities that informed subsequent tolerance and guidance strategies. Although no dedicated fatigue rig was employed, extended in-use exposure indicates adequate wear resistance and functional durability under realistic tremor-loading conditions.

4.5 Clinical Relevance

Functional performance was assessed through repeated execution of daily tasks with and without lock engagement. In the locked condition, visible tremor during eating and handwriting was reduced relative to the unlocked state, and task execution was more repeatable with fewer interruptions caused by involuntary motion. These findings support the clinical relevance of the proposed orthosis and motivate future studies using quantitative motion capture and standardized outcome measures.

5 Discussion

This section interprets numerical and experimental findings, benchmarks the proposed orthosis against existing solutions, and outlines refinements required for clinical translation. Quantitative values and uncertainties refer to Table 3.

5.1 Numerical and Experimental Findings

Numerical and experimental results were consistent, with global stiffness governed by the locking mechanism and the PLA shell acting as a compliant carrier. Total deformation reached (0.30 ± 0.02) mm for the 316 L configuration and (0.41 ± 0.03) mm for SLA, while engagement rod deflection was (0.038 ± 0.002) mm and (0.35 ± 0.03) mm, respectively. Stresses and contact pressures remained below material limits, yielding minimum safety factors above 1.8 for 316 L and approximately 1.1 for SLA, with numerical repeatability within ±5%.

Experimental testing confirmed robustness under handling and drop events. The assembled mass of (105 ± 3) g represents a 60–70% reduction compared with typical commercial wrist braces. User evaluation demonstrated stable tremor suppression in the locked state and preserved voluntary motion when unlocked, with only minor skin irritation after prolonged wear. Dimensional deviations at critical interfaces remained within ±0.1 mm.

5.2 Comparison with Existing Orthoses

Commercial wrist orthoses typically comprise soft braces enforcing continuous immobilization, hinged polymer braces restricting motion in a single plane, or active and semi-active systems that rely on sensors and actuators at the expense of increased mass and complexity. In contrast, the proposed device enables selective mechanical locking only when required, preserving unrestricted motion during routine use. The defined mechanical interface provides a repeatable end-stop with substantially higher engagement stiffness than strap-based polymer braces. While active systems can attenuate tremor, they introduce power, maintenance, and control burdens; the present passive design achieves comparable stabilization with significantly lower mass and no electronics. Whereas reported stiffness values for semi-rigid commercial braces typically range from 2–5 kN/mm, the mixed-material lock–shell configuration achieved approximately 9–10 kN/mm.

5.3 Limitations and Future Refinement

Although the orthosis met its mechanical and ergonomic objectives, further refinement is required before extended clinical deployment. Magnetic aids enabled coarse positioning but did not ensure repeatable alignment, occasionally increasing donning effort and load variability; passive alignment features such as keyed rails or tapered guides are therefore required to improve repeatability and reduce donning time below 20 s. Localized skin irritation after prolonged wear indicates the need for improved interface materials, while dimensional variability in SLA-printed bores highlights the importance of controlled locking-seat geometry via post-machined datum features or inserts. Static safety factors were sufficient, but cyclic durability remains unquantified, requiring long-term testing under representative tremor cycles (≥250 k cycles); measurement uncertainties of ±0.1 mm (geometry) and ±5% (loads) did not affect interpretation.

5.4 Implications for Clinical Translation

These results demonstrate that a passive, purely mechanical locking mechanism can deliver effective tremor stabilization while remaining lightweight, simple, and manufacturable. The mixed-material architecture supports low-cost, patient-specific orthoses producible via distributed additive manufacturing. Further clinical validation, durability testing, and ergonomic refinement are required to advance the system toward routine use in tremor and post-stroke rehabilitation.

6 Conclusions and Future Research

This work demonstrates a modular, purely mechanical wrist orthosis for selective tremor stabilization without electronics. Patient-specific scanning, parametric CAD, and additive manufacturing enabled a compact design with ergonomic fit and repeatable locking. Finite element analysis showed that the 316 L locking mechanism achieved high stiffness with low deformation ($\sim$0.30 mm) and a safety factor above 1.85, while SLA enabled rapid prototyping at reduced stiffness; prototype evaluation by a post-stroke participant confirmed functional stabilization, acceptable comfort, and agreement with numerical predictions.

Future work will focus on passive alignment guidance to simplify donning, improved comfort through optimized padding and ventilation, and long-term fatigue and wear studies, while exploring adjustable stiffness concepts that preserve passive reliability. The presented workflow demonstrates that patient-specific mechanical tuning enabled by additive manufacturing can provide effective tremor suppression without sensors, electronics, or external power.

References

1. Rocon E et al (2008) Wearable upper limb robots. In: Wearable robots, pp 235–281
2. Kotovsky J, Rosen MJ (1998) A wearable tremor-suppression orthosis. J Rehabil Res Dev 35(4):373–387
3. Takanokura M, Sugahara R, Miyake N, Ishiguro K, Muto T, Sakamoto K (2011) Upper-limb orthoses implemented with air dashpots for suppression of pathological tremor in daily activites
4. Hellwig B, Mund P, Schelter B, Guschlbauer B, Timmer J, Lücking CH (2009) A longitudinal study of tremor frequencies in Parkinson's disease and essential tremor. Clin Neurophysiol 120:431–435
5. Fromme NP, Camenzind M, Riener R, Rossi RM (2020) Design of a lightweight passive orthosis for tremor suppression. J Neuroeng Rehabil 17:47
6. Grimaldi G, Manto M (2010) "Old" and emerging therapies of human tremor. Clin. Med. Insights 2:CMT.S2999
7. Louis ED, Ferreira JJ (2010) How common is the most common adult movement disorder? Update on the worldwide prevalence of essential tremor. Mov Disord 25:534–541
8. Raghavan P (2015) Upper limb motor impairment after stroke. Phys Med Rehabil Clin N Am 26:599–610
9. Bansil S et al (2012) Movement disorders after stroke in adults: A review. Tremor Other Hyperkinet Mov (N. Y.) 2:tre–02–42–195–1
10. Samra E, Roushdy T, Zaki AS, Mansour AH, Elbassiouny A, Shalash A (2025) Frequency, phenotypes, and neuroimaging of early post stroke movement disorders: a prospective study. Egypt J Neurol Psychiatr Neurosurg 61:11

11. Miller KM, Okun MS, Fernandez HF, Jacobson CE t, Rodriguez RL, Bowers D (2007) Depression symptoms in movement disorders: comparing Parkinson's disease, dystonia, and essential tremor. Mov Disord 22:666–672
12. Rana AQ, Chou KL (2015) Clinical approach to essential tremor. In: Rana AQ, Chou KL (eds) Essential tremor in clinical practice. Springer International Publishing, Cham, pp 21–30
13. Pigg AC et al (2020) Distribution of tremor among the major degrees of freedom of the upper limb in subjects with essential tremor. Clin Neurophysiol 131:2700–2712
14. Charles SK, Hogan N (2011) Dynamics of wrist rotations. J Biomech 44:614–621
15. Taheri B, Case D, Richer E (2012) Design and development of a human arm joint simulator for evaluation of active assistive devices control algorithms. In: Adaptive control; advanced vehicle propulsion systems; aerospace systems; autonomous systems; battery modeling; biochemical systems; control over networks; control systems design; Cooperativ, vol 1. ASME, (Fort Lauderdale, Florida, USA), pp 707–714
16. Xu Y, Hollerbach J (1999) A robust ensemble data method for identification of human joint mechanical properties during movement. IEEE Trans Biomed Eng 46:409–419
17. Lakie M, Vernooij CA, Osborne TM, Reynolds RF (2012) The resonant component of human physiological hand tremor is altered by slow voluntary movements. J Physiol 590:2471–2483
18. Formica D, Charles SK, Zollo L, Guglielmelli E, Hogan N, Krebs HI (2012) The passive stiffness of the wrist and forearm. J Neurophysiol 108:1158–1166
19. Taheri B, Case D, Richer E (2014) Robust controller for tremor suppression at musculoskeletal level in human wrist. IEEE Trans Neural Syst Rehabil Eng 22:379–388
20. Case D, Taheri B, Richer E (2011) Dynamic magnetorheological damper for orthotic tremor suppression
21. Case D, Taheri B, Richer E (2015) Active control of MR wearable robotic orthosis for pathological tremor suppression. In: Multiagent network systems; natural gas and heat exchangers; path planning and motion control; powertrain systems; rehab robotics; robot manipulators; rollover prevention (AVS); sensors and actuators; time delay systems; tracking control systems; uncertain systems and robustness; un-manned, ground and surface robotics; vehicle dynamics control; vibration and control of smart structures/mech systems; vibration issues in mechanical systems, vol 3, American Society of Mechanical Engineers, Columbus, Ohio, USA
22. Katz R, Buki E, Zacksenhouse M (2017) Attenuating tremor using passive devices. Stud Health Technol Inform 242:741–747
23. Buki E, Katz R, Zacksenhouse M, Schlesinger I (2018) Vib-bracelet: a passive absorber for attenuating forearm tremor. Med Biol Eng Comput 56:923–930
24. Huen D, Liu J, Lo B (2016) An integrated wearable robot for tremor suppression with context aware sensing. In: 2016 IEEE 13th international conference on wearable and implantable body sensor networks (BSN). IEEE, (San Francisco, CA, USA), pp 312–317
25. Rocon E, Gallego JÁ, Belda-Lois JM, Benito-León J, Pons JL (2012) Biomechanical loading as an alternative treatment for tremor: a review of two approaches. Tremor Other Hyperkinet Mov (N. Y.) 2:02–77–495–1
26. Herrnstadt G, Menon C (2013) On-off tremor suppression orthosis with electromagnetic brake. Int. J. Mech. Eng. Mechatron 1(2), 7–24 (2013). https://doi.org/10.11159/ijmem.2013.002
27. Fromme NP (2022) Towards wearable tremor suppression orthoses. PhD thesis, ETH Zurich
28. Herrnstadt G, Menon C (2017) Elbow orthosis for tremor suppression – a torque based input case. In: Rojas I, Ortuño F (eds) Bioinformatics and biomedical engineering. Springer International Publishing, Cham, pp 292–302
29. Seki M et al (2011) Development of robotic upper limb orthosis with tremor suppressiblity and elbow joint movability. In: 2011 IEEE international conference on systems, man, and cybernetics. IEEE, Anchorage, AK, USA, pp 729–735

30. Matsumoto Y et al (2014) Development of an elbow-forearm interlock joint mechanism toward an exoskeleton for patients with essential tremor. In: 2014 IEEE/RSJ international conference on intelligent robots and systems. IEEE, Chicago, IL, USA, pp 2055–2062
31. Pons JL, Ceres R, Calderón L (2008) Introduction to wearable robotics. In: Wearable robots, pp 1–16
32. Kalaiarasi A, Kumar LA (2018) Sensor based portable tremor suppression device for stroke patients. Acupunct Electrother Res 43:29–37
33. Loureiro RCV, Belda-Lois JM, Lima ER, Pons JL, Sanchez-Lacuesta JJ, Harwin WS (2005) Upper limb tremor suppression in ADL via an orthosis incorporating a controllable double viscous beam actuator. In: 9th international conference on rehabilitation robotics, 2005. ICORR 2005, pp 119–122
34. van der Stelt M et al (2020) Improving lives in three dimensions: the feasibility of 3D printing for creating personalized medical aids in a rural area of Sierra Leone. Am. J. Trop. Med. Hyg. 102:905–909
35. Stoppa M, Chiolerio A (2014) Wearable electronics and smart textiles: a critical review. Sensors 14(7):11957–11992
36. Chen D, Pei Q (2017) Electronic muscles and skins: a review of soft sensors and actuators. Chem Rev 117:11239–11268
37. Fauland G, Lenz A, Rohrer C, Bechtold T (2013) Assessment of moisture management performance of multilayer compression bandages. Text Res J 83:871–880
38. Motlogelwa S (2018) Comfort and durability in high-performance clothing. In: High-performance apparel. Elsevier, pp 209–219
39. Lakie M, Vernooij CA, Osler CJ, Stevenson AT, Scott JPR, Reynolds RF (2015) Increased gravitational force reveals the mechanical, resonant nature of physiological tremor. J Physiol 593:4411–4422

Design and Manufacturing Workflow of a Patient-Specific Head Orthosis: A Case Study

A. Mrozek-Czajkowska[1(✉)], Wiesław Kuczko[1], M. Karolak[2], and J. Rybarczyk[1]

[1] Faculty of Mechanical Engineering, Poznan University of Technology, Piotrowo 3, 60-965 Poznań, Poland
agata.mrozek-czajkowska@put.poznan.pl
[2] The Feliks Nowowiejski Academy of Music, Slowackiego 7, 85-008 Bydgoszcz, Poland

Abstract. Recent advances in reverse engineering, surface scanning, and additive manufacturing have significantly expanded the capabilities of modern orthopaedics, enabling the development of highly individualized orthotic devices. While cranial orthoses are traditionally associated with pediatric applications, their potential extends to adult patients requiring post-traumatic, postoperative, or neurological support. Essential Tremor (ET), one of the most common movement disorders, often progresses to involve cranial structures, creating a need for customized head-stabilizing solutions. In this work, a patient-specific head orthosis was designed and fabricated to provide stabilization while maintaining controlled transverse head rotation. The design workflow incorporated handheld 3D scanning, digital reconstruction using a scaled open-source cranial model, and modeling of orthotic components. Two interface variants—a rigid configuration and a flexible configuration incorporating TPU—were developed to evaluate structural and ergonomic performance. The orthosis components were manufactured using Fused Deposition Modeling (FDM) with TPU and PLA Pro materials, followed by post-processing and integration of EVA foam for improved comfort. A neoprene orthopedic corset and carbon-fiber support rods ensured stable attachment to the torso. The final prototype demonstrates the feasibility of producing lightweight, functional, and anatomically tailored orthoses for ET patients. Potential future enhancements include embedding pressure sensors for internal load monitoring and adaptive, sensor driven control of device stiffness.

Keywords: Essential Tremor · Head Orthosis · Additive Manufacturing

1 Introduction

In recent years, the field of orthopaedics has experienced substantial advancements, driven, among others, by progress in reverse engineering and rapid prototyping technologies. These developments have enabled the creation of highly individualized orthopaedic devices, including orthoses and prostheses, offering enhanced comfort, functionality, and improved adaptation to patient-specific injuries [1–5].

F. Górski et al. (Eds.): MANUFACTURING 2026, LNME, pp. 115–127, 2026.
https://doi.org/10.1007/978-3-032-23089-8_10

Head orthoses are most commonly associated with cranial remolding orthoses used for infants with skull deformities such as plagiocephaly [6, 7]. Early cranial deformities may lead to long-term health and aesthetic consequences in a developing child. Individualized helmet therapy is intended to guide the skull toward a healthy growth pattern; however, not every helmet geometry ensures an optimal therapeutic outcome. To achieve proper fit and effectiveness, a scanning procedure based on a handheld surface scanner was evaluated to accurately capture the patient's cranial morphology [8, 9].

Although the pediatric application of head orthoses is the most widely recognized, the potential use of individualized cranial orthoses is not limited to infants. This type of orthopaedic appliance is also used in post-traumatic, postoperative, and neurological cases in which precise support, stabilization, or protection of cranial structures is required. A 3D-printed helmet provides a widely accessible and safe protective solution for patients undergoing for example decompressive craniectomy [10].

In the study [11] by Kropla et al., an alternative workflow for helmet fabrication was introduced, utilizing a non-invasive surface 3D scan (Artec Leo, Artec3D). This approach enables precise acquisition of cranial metrics, individualized helmet design, and direct comparison with routinely obtained CT scans. All enrolled patients underwent a surface 3D scan, after which a customized helmet was fabricated to cover the craniectomy site. The study demonstrated that non-invasive 3D scanning represents a feasible, accurate, and clinically practical method for assessing cranial geometry after DC and for guiding the construction of 3D-printed protective helmets [11].

Another condition overcome with head orthoses is Dropped Head Syndrome, a passively correctable cervical deformity. Recent work has explored mobile cervical orthoses that stabilize the head while maintaining neck mobility, thereby improving user comfort and quality of life. Passive designs are particularly promising due to their simplicity and compact form, although ensuring sufficient support remains a challenge. In this context, the study by Torrendell et al. [12] proposed a novel compliant mechanism designed to provide adjustable and non-restrictive assistance during anterior and posterior neck flexion while preserving unrestricted axial rotation. Their experimental evaluation in healthy participants indicated that the device effectively offloaded the cervical musculature without inducing compensatory overload and maintained free rotation across all tested stiffness configurations.

In the development of neurodegenerative diseases, the phenomenon of neuronal loss is observed. The resulting symptoms of neurological damage can be assigned to two main groups: those related to memory disorders and those related to motor function disorders. Motor dysfunctions manifest primarily as tremor. Tremor consists of involuntary rhythmic movements caused by rhythmic contractions of antagonistic muscles. The clinical classification of tremor depends on its location, the position in which the tremor amplitude is greatest, and the tremor frequency [13]. The classification of tremor based on frequency includes dividing it into specific frequency bands associated with particular disorders. Tremor frequencies occurring in essential tremor (ET), predominantly during action, range from 8 to 12 Hz [14, 15]. This is one of the most common disorders of this type alongside Parkinson's disease.

Tremors that occur during intentional activities like writing or eating usually affect the hands and arms, but over time can spread to the head (neck area), voice, jaw, and other parts of the body [16]. Due to this fact, a procedure of designing and manufacturing was developed to create individual head stabilizing orthoses specifically designed for this type of disorder.

2 Research Problem

An essential feature of the head orthosis was its personalization to the individual patient. The primary task of the orthosis was to provide stabilization while allowing small movements—specifically, rotation of the head in the transverse plane. The proposed orthosis-modeling workflow is shown in Fig. 1.

The procedure began with the measurement of the patient's head circumference, followed by the acquisition of the upper-back and partial cranial geometry using a handheld EinScan Pro 3D scanner. Although the scanner provided accurate reconstruction of the exposed anatomical regions, the presence of hair prevented the capture of the complete cranial surface, resulting in missing geometric data in the superior and lateral areas of the head (Fig. 2a).

To address this limitation, a reference head model obtained from an open-source repository [17] was integrated into the workflow. The generic model was scaled according to the measured head circumference and subsequently aligned with the available scan data (Fig. 2b, c). The positioning process was further refined by matching distinctive anatomical features present in the scan—most notably the auricular structures—to ensure consistency between the digital reconstruction and the patient's anatomy.

Following the generation of a complete head geometry, 3D sketches were created directly on the reconstructed surface and used as the basis for orthosis modeling. The head-encircling component of the orthosis was designed as two interconnected segments. All sketches and solid features were developed using Autodesk Inventor 2025. In Fig. 3, the two principal sketches are highlighted, with one displayed in red and the other in yellow to clearly distinguish the functional elements of the design.

The thickness of the head-encircling component was defined as 6 mm, which ensured sufficient structural stiffness while maintaining a lightweight profile suitable for patient comfort (Fig. 4). An initial prototype of this component was manufactured and fitted to the patient to verify the accuracy of the head-model scaling and the overall geometrical conformity. The fitting procedure confirmed the correct alignment of the orthosis with key anatomical landmarks, enabling the continuation of the design process for the remaining components of the system.

Following the preliminary fitting stage, a uniform 4 mm offset was introduced on the inner surface of the head-encircling model to include an EVA foam layer, intended to improve comfort, reduce localized pressure, and enhance stability during use. The implementation of this offset was essential for ensuring proper integration of the soft interface material without compromising the functional geometry of the orthosis.

After designing the head-encircling component, the remaining elements of the orthosis had to be defined to ensure both mobility and adequate stabilization of the patient. For this purpose, two carbon-fiber flat bars with a cross-section of 6×15 mm were selected. The length of each bar was customized according to the patient's anthropometric dimensions—specifically, the vertical distance from the most prominent point of the

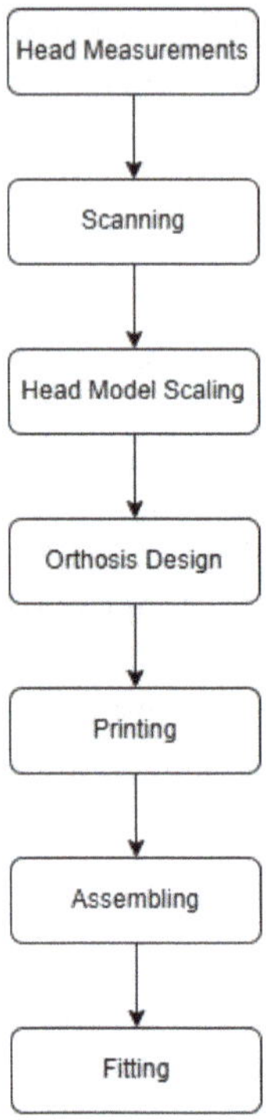

Fig. 1. Workflow of the design and manufacturing process of the head orthosis

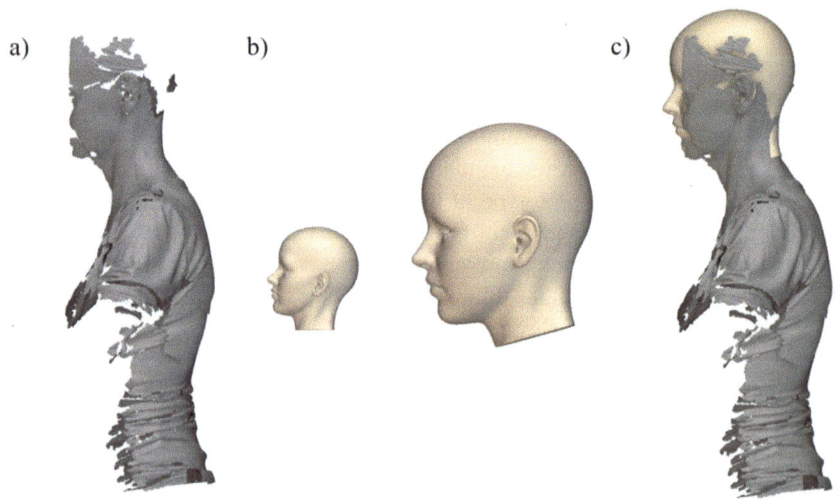

Fig. 2. Steps of obtaining the head geometry: a) geometry captured during 3D scanning, b) scaling of the full head model to the patient's dimensions, c) final result of fitting the head model to the scan.

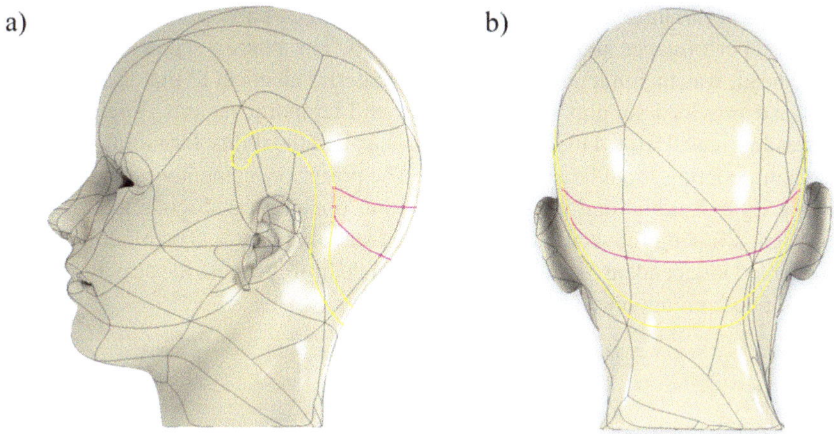

Fig. 3. Created orthosis sketches: a) lateral view, b) posterior view

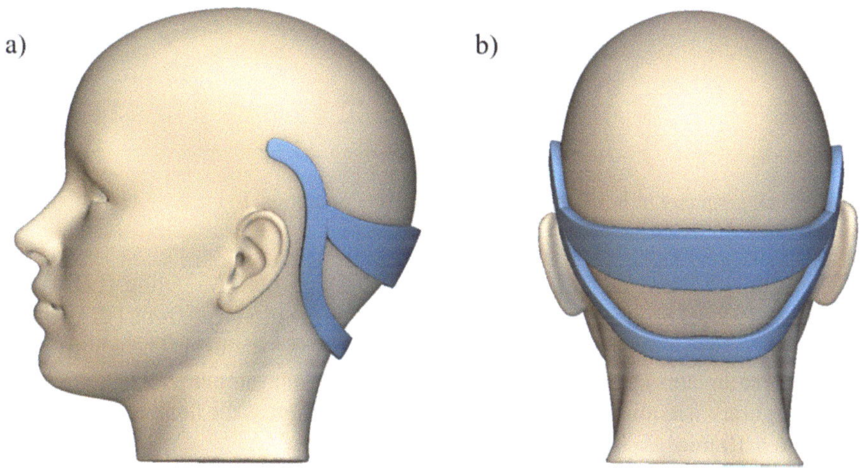

Fig. 4. Final geometry of head-encircling component: a) lateral view, b) posterior view

skull to approximately the level of the sacrum. To ensure stable attachment of the bars to the patient's torso, an orthopedic corset was incorporated into the design.

Figure 5 presents two variants of the head–orthosis interface designed to connect the cranial component with the stabilizing support rods. The first variant (Fig. 5a) characterized a single-material structure in which the head-encircling component and the rod-mounting extension are manufactured as one rigid part. This extension incorporated press-fit insertion openings located on the underside of the element, enabling secure attachment of the stabilizing rods. To prevent accidental detachment, the rods were additionally retained using a magnetic strap mechanism. This solution provided high structural stiffness, although it limits local compliance.

The second variant (Fig. 5b) employed a modular, three-part configuration to improve mechanical performance and enhance user comfort. The anterior segment, which encircled the head, was manufactured from a rigid material identical to that used in the first variant and provided support in the occipital and temporal regions. The central segment was fabricated from TPU, introducing controlled flexibility for vibration damping and accommodating small head movements. The posterior segment was produced from the same rigid material and contained mounting openings analogous to those in the first design, allowing for secure insertion of the stabilizing rods. The modular arrangement enabled independent tuning of stiffness and flexibility across the structure, thereby improving both ergonomics and adjustability.

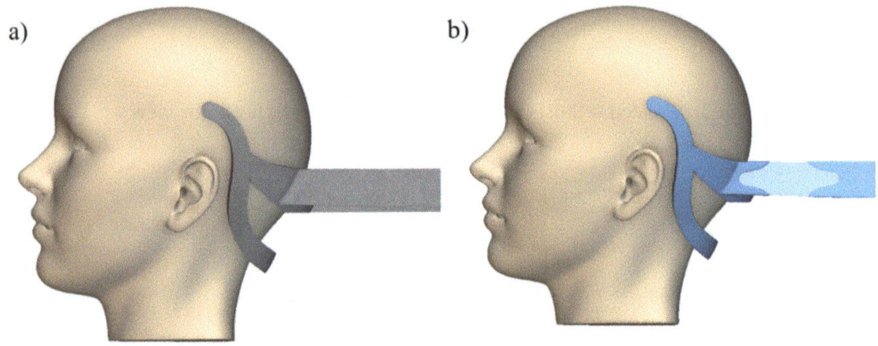

Fig. 5. Final geometry of head orthosis: a) the rigid configuration, b) the flexible configuration

The orthoses were manufactured using Fused Deposition Modeling (FDM) on a Bambu Lab P1S 3D printer. The flexible components were produced from TPU, whereas the rigid elements were fabricated using Spectrum PLA Pro filament. The additive manufacturing parameters applied in the fabrication process are summarized in Table 1. The rigid configuration required 7 h 2 min of printing time, whereas the flexible configuration required 6 h 10 min.

Table 1. Additive manufacturing parameters

	Material	
Property	TPU	PLA Pro
layer height [mm]	0.28	0.20
infill [%]	5	15
nozzle temperature [°C]	230	260

The designed prototype was also tested using the Finite Element Method (FEM) to assess the safety of its application for the patient. The analysis was conducted in the Abaqus 2022 environment. The created rigid configuration prototype model was discretized using tetrahedral C3D10 elements. The applied finite element mesh consisted of 189,203 nodes and 99,090 elements (Fig. 6). The material properties were defined based on the manufacturer's Technical Data Sheet [18]. Young's modulus was 2,865 MPa and the tensile strength was equal to 40 MPa.

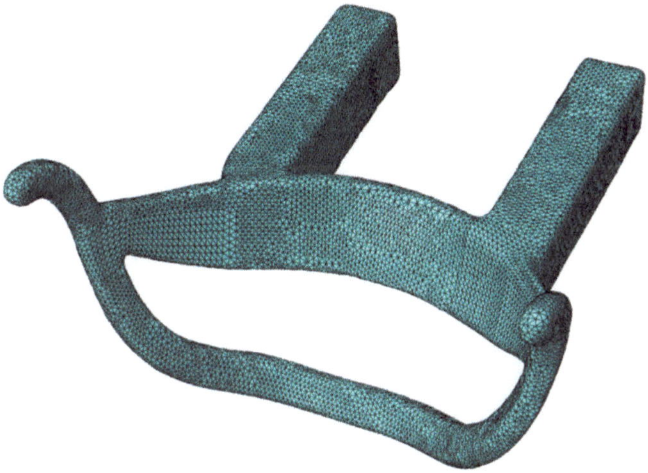

Fig. 6. Applied finite element mesh

The defined boundary conditions included a fixed constraint at the orthosis attachment location to the stabilizing rods (Fig. 7). In addition, a pressure load was applied on the contact surface between the head and the orthosis, based on the study [19], in which average and peak pressures were recorded for eight participants during three selected tasks: walking, running, and kneeling forward. In the analysis, a worst-case load corresponding to the maximum recorded peak pressure (0.024 MPa) was applied.

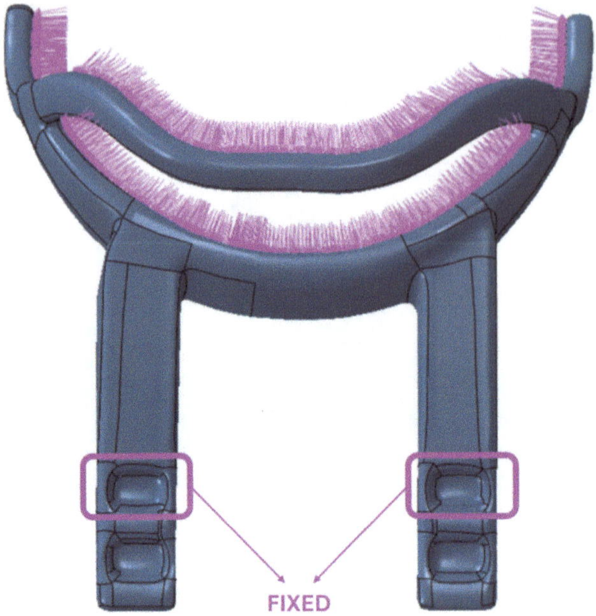

Fig. 7. Load and boundary conditions

3 Results

The parameters applied during the additive manufacturing process enabled the correct fabrication of the orthosis geometry. The fabricated components required post-processing, including support removal, surface grinding, and elimination of sharp or protruding material residues. The components obtained directly after the printing process are presented in Figs. 8 and 9. After post-processing, the internal surfaces of the orthoses were lined with EVA foam.

The foam was bonded to the inner surfaces of the orthosis using waterproof double-sided adhesive tape. The foam layer filled the offset intentionally introduced during the design stage, ensuring proper cushioning and improved user comfort (Fig. 10).

The Fig. 11 presents the final configuration of the orthosis, in which the flexible and rigid versions are interchangeable. To ensure stable attachment of the stabilizing bars to the patient's torso, a commercial orthopedic corset was incorporated into the design (manufacturer: TOROS-GROUP). Due to the stiffness of the molded ribs and the structural characteristics of the thoracic region, the corset provided stabilization of both the thoracic and lumbar spine. The wide shoulder straps distributed pressure evenly across the shoulders, while the waist straps delivered the required level of compression and fixation, thereby reducing discomfort in the upper and lower spinal regions. The corset was made of neoprene.

FEM results indicated that the orthosis was predominantly subjected to low stress levels, with values below 5 MPa. Noticeable stress values occurred locally around the geometric connection zone (Fig. 12). The highest stresses were concentrated at the junction between the straight segment of the orthosis connected to the stabilizing rods

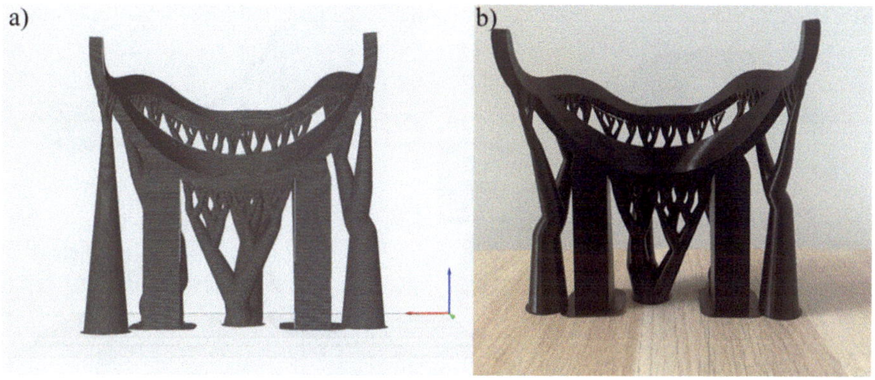

Fig. 8. Rigid configuration: a) visualization of the manufacturing process in Bambu Studio, b) component after the manufacturing process

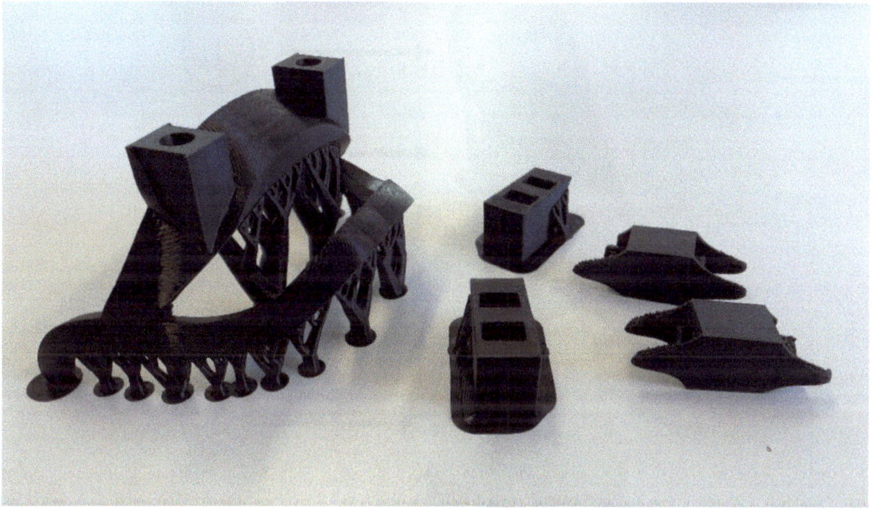

Fig. 9. Components after the manufacturing process – flexible configuration

and the curved supporting head element, particularly at the inner corner, where a peak value of 30 MPa was observed. These values did not exceed the allowable limits.

A similar pattern was visible in the maximum principal logarithmic strain distribution (Fig. 13). The maximum strain reached 0.53%, confirming that the deformation was highly localized near the geometric discontinuity. In the remaining parts of the orthosis, strain values were significantly lower.

a)

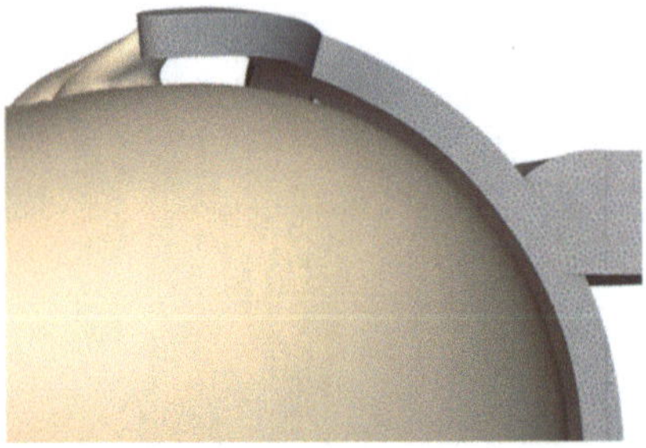

b)

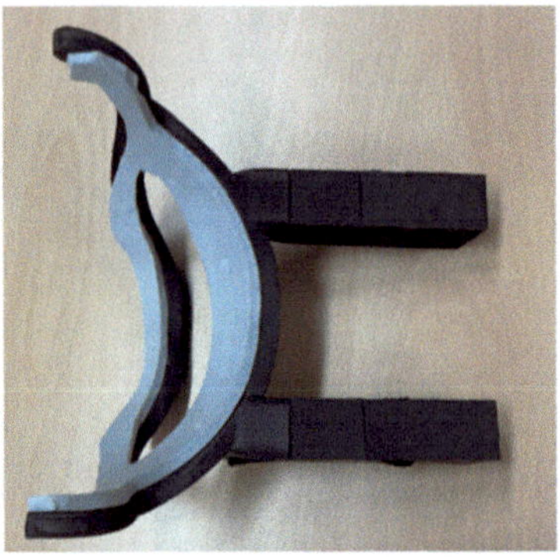

Fig. 10. Final configuration of the head-encircling component: a) visualization of the designed offset, b) component with the EVA foam attached

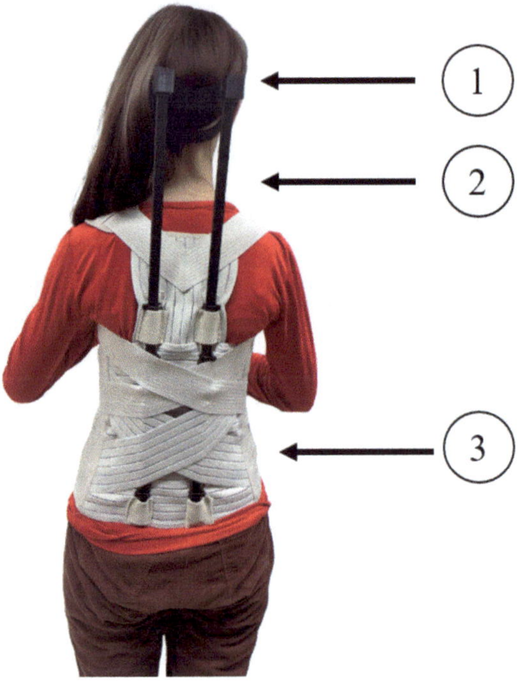

Fig. 11. View of the assembled orthosis: 1 – 3D-printed orthosis, 2 – stabilizing rods, 3 – mounting corset

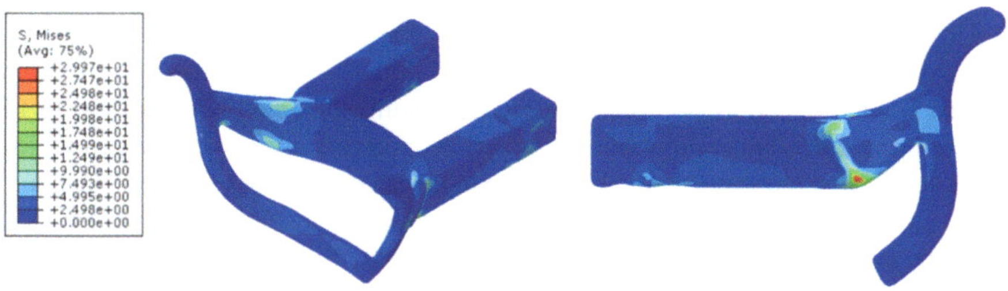

Fig. 12. Von Mises stress distribution map [MPa]

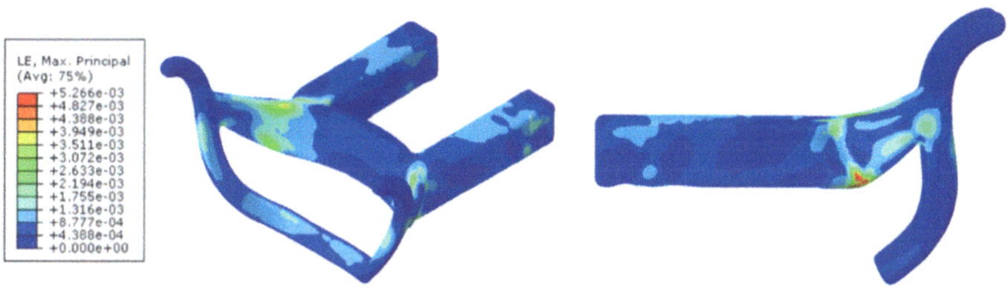

Fig. 13. Logarithmic strain distribution [–]

4 Discussion

The developed orthosis primarily provides stabilization for individuals affected ET, while the flexible configuration additionally enables a controlled range of head rotation in the transverse plane. The geometry of the device was fully customized to the patient, ensuring proper anatomical compatibility and improved comfort during use. The orthosis remained lightweight, functional, and sufficiently mobile to adapt to the user's daily activities while maintaining the required level of support.

The loads used in the FEM analysis were adopted based on existing studies that recorded the pressure between the head and the helmet during selected activities such as running, walking, and forward kneeling. For further optimization of the orthosis design, the integration of pressure sensors in the proposed orthosis designs could be considered. These sensors could be embedded at anatomically relevant locations, enabling the acquisition of patient-specific pressure distribution data at the interface between the orthosis and the patient, tailored to the individual and the stage of disease progression.

In addition, permanently embedded sensors could provide continuous information regarding changes in the patient's condition. Long-term data acquisition would support monitoring the progression of ET and could facilitate the development of a future mechatronic orthosis capable of adapting its stiffness or damping characteristics to the patient's tremor frequency and intensity in real time. Such an adaptive system would represent an advanced step toward personalized, responsive assistive devices for individuals with movement disorders.

5 Conclusions

The proposed head orthosis provides effective stabilization for individuals with ET while offering a flexible configuration that permits controlled transverse head rotation. The patient-specific design ensured proper anatomical conformity, comfort, and functional usability, whereas additive manufacturing enabled lightweight yet durable components. The modular construction allows for interchangeability between rigid and flexible variants, adapting the device to individual therapeutic needs.

Future enhancements may include the integration of pressure sensors to monitor internal load distribution, support finite element–based structural optimization, and enable long-term tracking of disease progression. Such developments could ultimately lead to a next-generation adaptive mechatronic orthosis capable of dynamically responding to tremor characteristics, further improving patient support and quality of life.

Acknowledgments. This research was funded by the grant 0612/SBAD/3642, Funded by the Ministry of Science and Higher Education, Poland. Part of the studies were realized in scope of the grant entitled "Biomedical Innovations through Digital Transformation of Additive Technologies and Knowledge Exchange – BIOMEDIX" supported by ERASMUS+ (2024-1-LV01-KA220-HED-000255929).

References

1. Górski F (2025) Computer aided design of 3D printable anatomically shaped medical devices: methodologies and applications, 1st edn. CRC Press, Boca Raton
2. Górski F et al (2025) Automation of design of modular upper limb prostheses. Facta Universitatis, Series: Mechanical Engineering. University of Niš, Serbia
3. Jańczak K, Górski F, Żukowska M, Rybarczyk J, Barteczka T, Kuczko W (2025) The application of additive manufacturing technology in designing and producing individualized lower limb orthoses. Adv Sci Technol Res J 19(7):346–359
4. Górski F et al (2024) Individualized 3D printed orthopaedic and prosthetic devices using AutoMedPrint technology – methodologies and examples. Adv Sci Technol Res J 18(6):145–158
5. Górski F, Żukowska M, Wierzbicka N, Wichniarek R, Comsa D-S, Smolarek E (2025) Automated design of 3D printed biomedical products with use of knowledge-based engineering (KBE). In: W BIOMEDIX: advancing biomedical innovation through digital transformation. Zenodo
6. Kropla F, Hoffmann M, Winkler D et al (2023) Development of an individual helmet orthosis for infants based on a 3D scan. 3D Print Med 9:22
7. Kunz F et al (2019) Head orthosis therapy in positional plagiocephaly: longitudinal 3D-investigation of long-term outcomes compared with untreated infants and with a control group. Eur J Orthod 41(1):29–37
8. Atallah H et al (2025) Customized 3D printed helmet in the treatment of metopic craniosynostosis in a 7-month-old infant: case report. Front Pediatr 13:1474412
9. Atallah H et al (2025) 3D-printed cranial helmet therapy for the treatment of deformational plagiocephaly. Front Pediatr 13:1638581

10. Pang SSY, Fang E, Chen KW et al (2022) Patient-specific 3D-printed helmet for post-craniectomy defect – a case report. 3D Print Med 8:4
11. Kropla F, Wach J, Winkler D, Grunert R, Güresir E, Vychopen M (2025) Noninvasive 3D head scan used for 3D-printed customized helm in a patient undergoing decompressive hemicraniectomy. Front Bioeng Biotechnol 13:1530126
12. Torrendell SP, Kadone H, Hassan M, Chen Y, Miura K, Suzuki K (2024) A neck orthosis with multi-directional variable stiffness for persons with dropped head syndrome. IEEE Robot Autom Lett 9(7):6224–6231
13. Orzechowski T, Wochlik I (2011) Metody pomiaru i analizy sygnału drżenia i dysfunkcji ruchowych w chorobach neurodegeneracyjnych. Pomiary Automatyka Robotyka 15(12):116–120
14. Burne JA, Hayes MW, Fung VS, Yiannikas C, Boljevac D (2002) The contribution of tremor studies to the diagnosis of parkinsonian and essential tremor: a statistical evaluation. J Clin Neurosci 9:237–242
15. Cichaczewski E, Munhoz RP, Maia JM, Nohama P, Nóvak EM, Teive HA (2014) Electrophysiologic characteristics of tremor in Parkinson's disease and essential tremor. Arq Neuropsiquiatr 72(4):301–306
16. Louis ED, Gerbin M, Galecki M (2013) Essential tremor 10, 20, 30, 40: clinical snapshots of the disease by decade of duration. Eur J Neurol 20:949–954
17. Thingverse Homepage: https://www.thingiverse.com/thing:979818, Last accessed: 20 Nov 2025
18. Spectrum Filaments Homepage: https://spectrumfilaments.com/, Last accessed: 12 Jan 2026
19. Niu J, Zhang C, Chen X, Ma C, Chen L, Tong C (2019) A novel helmet fitness evaluation device based on the flexible pressure sensor matrix. Sensors 19(18):3823

Design and Investigation of a Low-Cost, Anatomically Customized Mechatronic Hand Prosthesis

J. Rybarczyk(✉), M. Dolatkowski, Filip Górski, A. Mrozek-Czajkowska, and P. Nowak

Poznan University of Technology, Poznań, Poland
justyna.rybarczyk@put.poznan.pl

Abstract. This article presents a comprehensive approach to the design and fabrication of an upper-limb prosthesis developed using a modular concept and generated through the AutoMedPrint system on the basis of high-resolution 3D scans of the patient's residual limb. Biomedical engineering, which integrates core engineering disciplines such as mechanics, electronics, chemistry, and optics, provides the methodological framework for creating advanced prosthetic devices aimed at restoring lost functionality by replacing absent or damaged biological structures. The clinical demand for functional upper-limb prostheses is particularly noticeable among young users, who often exhibit increased expectations regarding device speed, strength, ergonomics, and aesthetics. At the same time, the high rejection rates reported in paediatric and adolescent populations underline the importance of personalized and adaptable prosthetic solutions.

In the presented article, the digital prosthetic model was integrated with an electronic control system enabling functional actuation of the device. The structural components were produced using additive manufacturing technologies, ensuring high geometric accuracy, reduced production costs, and the possibility of rapid iteration during the design process. A detailed geometric analysis was carried out in a virtual environment, allowing verification of fit, structural correctness, and component interactions before physical fabrication. The objective of the study was to develop a cost-effective, patient-specific mechatronic prosthesis that meets the functional requirements of an adolescent user while addressing the broader challenges associated with long-term prosthesis acceptance.

Keywords: Additive Manufacturing · Hand Protestesis · AutoMedPrint

1 Introduction

Biomedical engineering integrates fundamental engineering disciplines—such as electronics, chemistry, optics, and mechanics—with medical technologies, providing, among other solutions, prosthetic devices that replace missing or damaged anatomical structures [1, 2]. In patients with congenital or acquired limb absence, impaired grasping ability significantly hinders the performance of daily activities, which creates a strong demand for effective upper-limb prosthetic solutions.

F. Górski et al. (Eds.): MANUFACTURING 2026, LNME, pp. 128–140, 2026.
https://doi.org/10.1007/978-3-032-23089-8_11

Despite technological progress, abandonment rates for prosthetic devices remain high, particularly within the pediatric population. According to the literature, 32–45% of children and 23–39% of adults discontinue the use of prostheses, depending on the type of device [3]. The intensive somatic development occurring between 0 and 21 years of age leads to recommendations favoring cosmetic or passive prostheses, which may limit later adaptation to active devices. Previous studies have shown that fitting a child with a prosthesis before the 30th month of life does not affect long-term functional competence [4], whereas introducing a myoelectric prosthesis at approximately 54 months significantly reduces the likelihood of rejection [5]. The most common periods of discontinuation for electrically powered prostheses occur before the 6th and 14th year of use, resulting respectively from operational difficulties or increasing functional expectations during adolescence [6]. Furthermore, previous experience with body-powered prostheses correlates with longer daily usage times of myoelectric devices, supporting the adaptation process [5].

The current market offers a limited number of certified myoelectric prostheses for children. Typical designs employ a single motor and silicone cosmetic gloves.

This article presents the design, fabrication, and evaluation of a mechatronic hand prosthesis prototype developed for a 15-year-old patient with congenital upper-limb deficiency. The patient has several years of experience using low-cost, body-powered prostheses manufactured with the AutoMedPrint technology. According to literature data, the patient's age profile is associated with a low risk of rejecting an electric prosthesis; however, it also entails high expectations regarding performance parameters such as grip force, actuation speed, and ergonomics. The subsequent sections of this article detail the implemented design solutions, the results of conducted analyses, and the functional evaluation of the developed prototype [7–10].

2 Research Problem

2.1 Aim of the Work

The aim of this study was to develop a functional, low-cost, fully personalized mechatronic upper limb prosthesis designed for a 15-year-old patient with congenital transradial amputation. A key design assumption was the integration of a modular model automatically generated in the AutoMedPrint environment with custom mechatronic components—particularly an active hand drive and a compact wrist rotation mechanism. The study sought to provide a procedure enabling rapid and precise fabrication of pediatric prostheses by combining the capabilities of additive manufacturing with Customize digital parameterization and functional evaluation.

2.2 AutoMedPrint System

AutoMedPrint is a system that enables the generation of anatomically fitted prosthetic models based on high-resolution 3D scans (as shown in Fig. 1). The system automates the creation of socket geometry and forearm segments, using 3D mesh processing methods and user-defined cutting planes [7, 10].

In this work, the system served as a starting point for further structural modifications—ensuring proper fit to the patient's residual limb and providing a supporting framework for the mechatronic components. The resulting model required local adjustments (collision elimination, wall thickness modification, addition of mounting spaces), which were introduced already at the design stage within the CAD environment [7, 10].

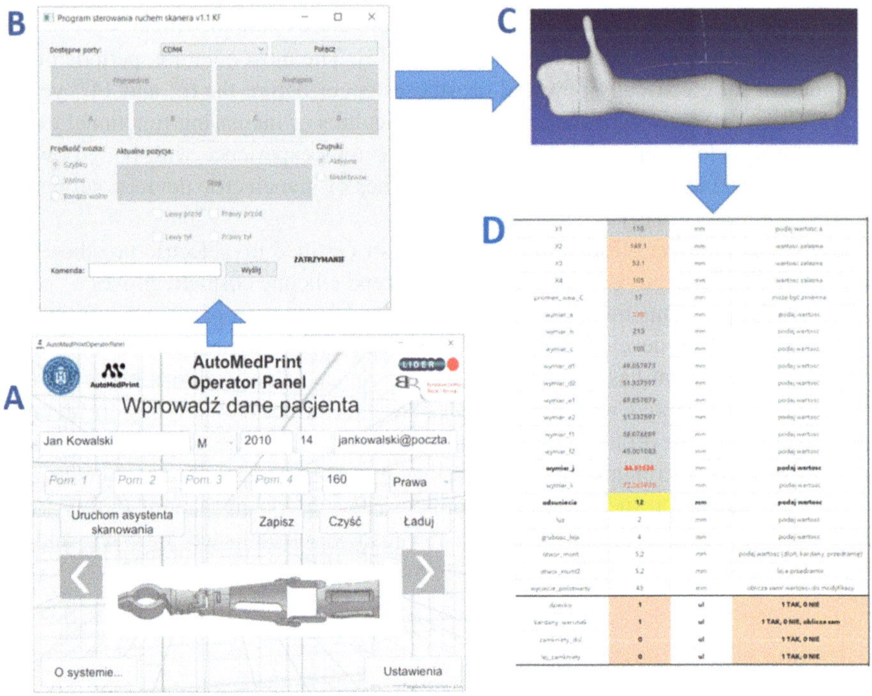

Fig. 1. The scheme of data processing: (a) AutoMedPrint Operator Panel Software; (b) control the movement of the scanner software; (c) scan processing software (MeshLab); (d) an automated Excel spreadsheet [10].

2.3 Material and Background

The prosthesis design was based on a combination of additive technology (FDM) and conventional machining. Structural models were produced from high-stiffness polymer filaments, while components requiring increased precision, dimensional stability, and mechanical strength (bushings, shafts, gear elements) were manufactured from metals (as shown in Fig. 2).

From a clinical perspective, the patient belonged to a group of users with a low risk of rejecting a myoelectric prosthesis, but at the same time with high demands regarding grip strength, operating speed, and ergonomics. The user's prior experience with prostheses made in AutoMedPrint enabled a proper comparative evaluation of the mechatronic solution's functionality [7].

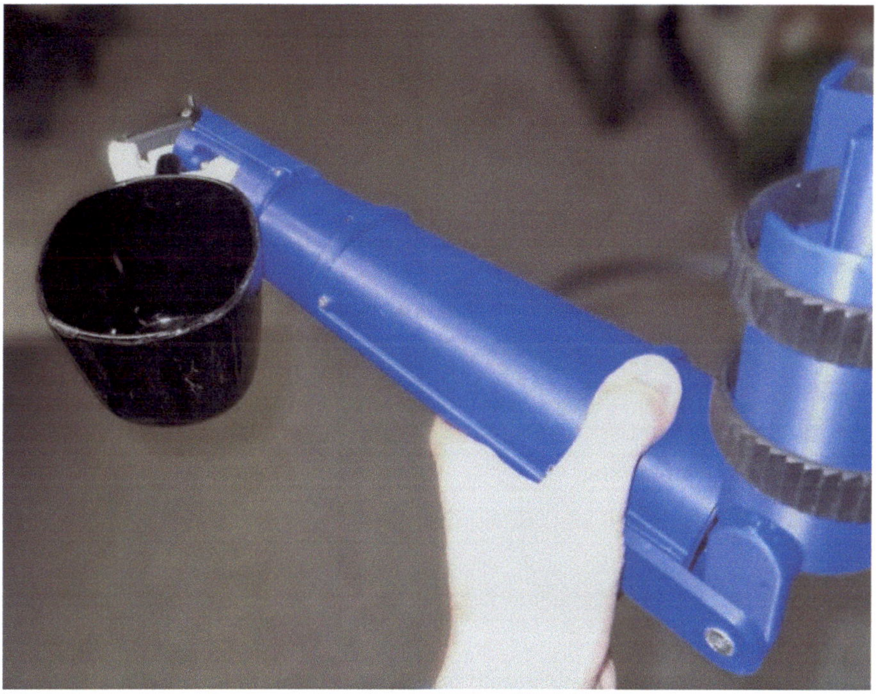

Fig. 2. Application of the prosthesis in performing the task of lifting a cup [7].

2.4 Design and Mechanical Development

The design process encompassed comprehensive activities aimed at integrating anatomical geometry with advanced mechatronic components. The starting point was the reconstruction of a healthy hand based on 3D scans and the creation of its mirrored counterpart, which allowed the proper proportions and shape of the limb to be reproduced. Subsequently, the baseline model generated by AutoMedPrint (shown in Fig. 3.) was imported into Autodesk Inventor 2024, where it underwent further modifications. At this stage, a structure was developed that enabled the installation of two compact drives—the hand-closing mechanism and active wrist rotation. Particular attention was devoted to minimizing the space required by the drive systems so that they could fit within the limited volume of the patient's forearm (shown in Fig. 4.) [7].

The hand mechanism was equipped with a motor coupled to a high-ratio gearbox, providing adequate gripping force. The wrist drive, in turn, was based on a self-locking transmission, ensuring positional stability without the need for continuous power supply. Within the CAD environment, the motion of all components was analyzed, collisions and assembly feasibility were verified, cable routing was examined, and structural stiffness was assessed. During the design process, a compartment was also developed to house the control electronics, including an FSR pressure sensor and an Arduino Nano microcontroller, responsible for operating the prosthesis based on the pressure force generated by the user [7]. An exploded view of the assembly, excluding the previously described elements, pressure sensors, and mounting components (for clarity), is shown in Fig. 5.

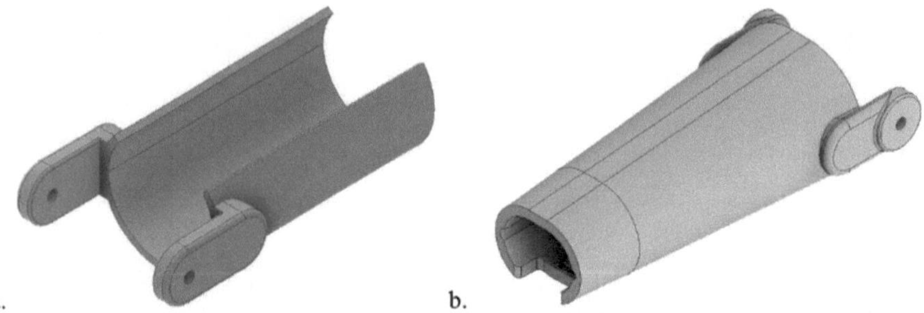

a. b.

Fig. 3. Models obtained using the AutoMedPrint system. a. – prosthetic socket, b. – forearm sect [7].

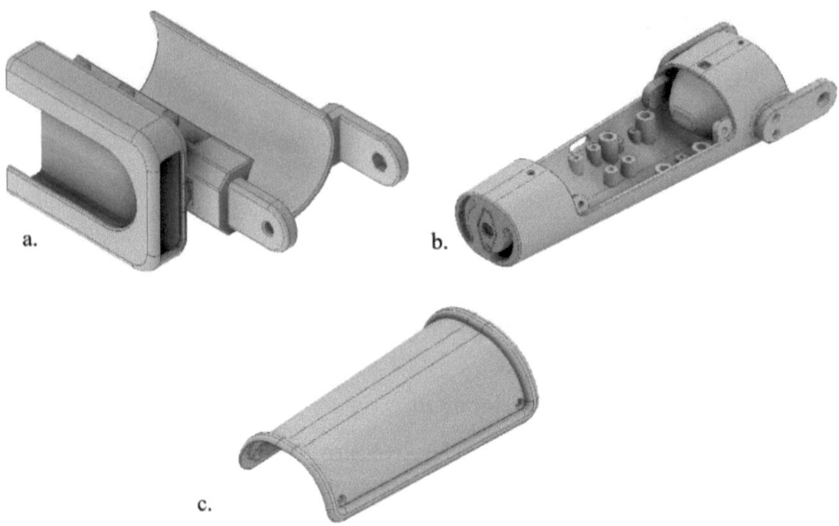

a. b. c.

Fig. 4. a. – prosthetic socket model adapted for the mechatronic design, b. – forearm model adapted for the mechatronic design, c. – forearm cover [7].

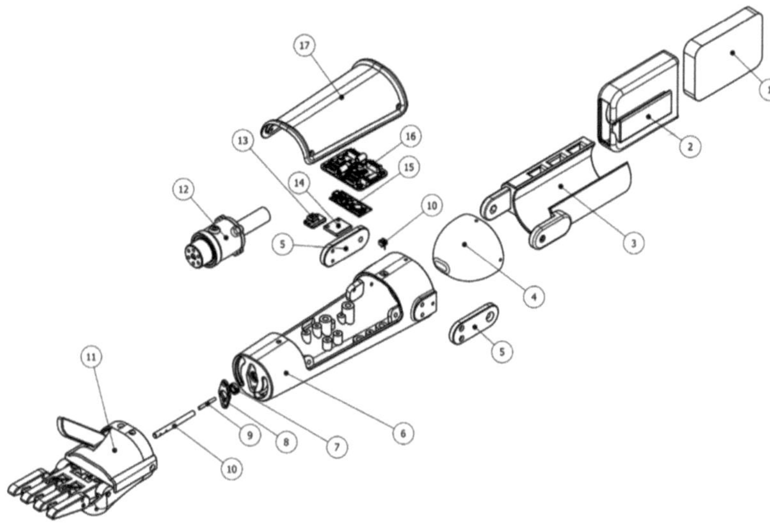

Fig. 5. Exploded view of the designed device. 1 – energy bank, 2 – energy bank basket, 3 – prosthetic funnel, 4 – funnel socket, 5 – forearm mounting wings, 6 – forearm, 7 – DIN 625 SKF bearing, 9 – wrist calibration lock, 10 – wrist drive shaft, 11 – hand prosthesis, 12 – wrist drive system, 13 – Adafruit 4090 module, 14 – bidirectional current, power, and voltage sensor based on the INA226 integrated circuit, 15 – Nano V3.0 board, 16 – Hiwonder four-channel motor controller with encoder, 17 – forearm cover [7].

3 Results

3.1 Manufacturing Results

The manufacturing process confirmed that the designed structure can be fully realized using **FFF technology** with PETG material, which provided favorable mechanical properties and adequate dimensional stability for all structural elements of the prosthesis. Owing to its higher stiffness and fracture resistance compared to PLA, PETG proved particularly well suited for prosthetic applications, where maintaining a balance between strength and flexibility in load-bearing zones is essential.

Components produced on Bambu Lab P1S, X1 Carbon, and H2D printers exhibited excellent dimensional repeatability and required no post-assembly adjustments. The high interlayer adhesion of PETG translated into sufficient rigidity of the hand, wrist, and forearm components, while simultaneously allowing the device to remain lightweight. The use of optimized printing parameters—primarily an increased number of perimeters, controlled infill, and moderate layer height—enabled the construction to withstand loads generated during grasping and rotational movements. The production process planning for all components of the forearm prosthesis module is shown in Fig. 6.

The application of PETG was particularly critical in areas requiring enhanced resistance to deformation, such as the hand casing and motor mounting spaces. The material demonstrated dimensional stability both during printing and after cooling, which significantly reduced the risk of warping and improved the quality of joints between polymer and metallic components.

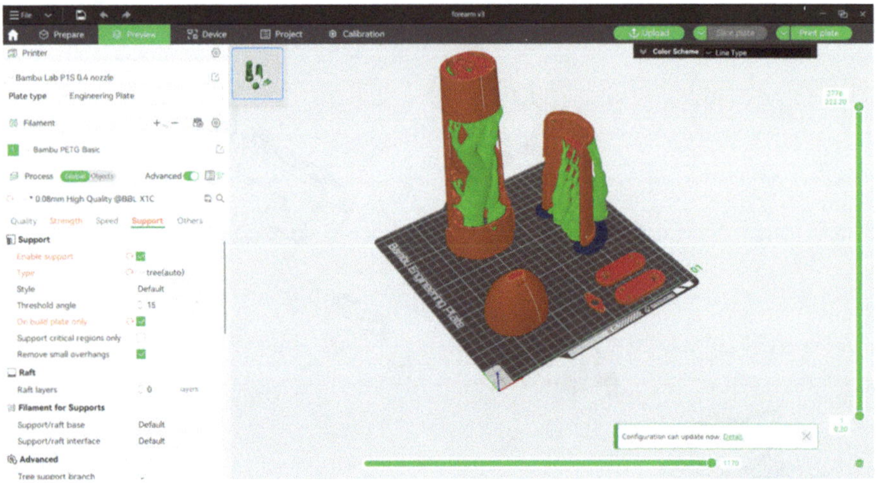

Fig. 6. Planning the manufacturing process for all components of the prosthetic forearm module [7].

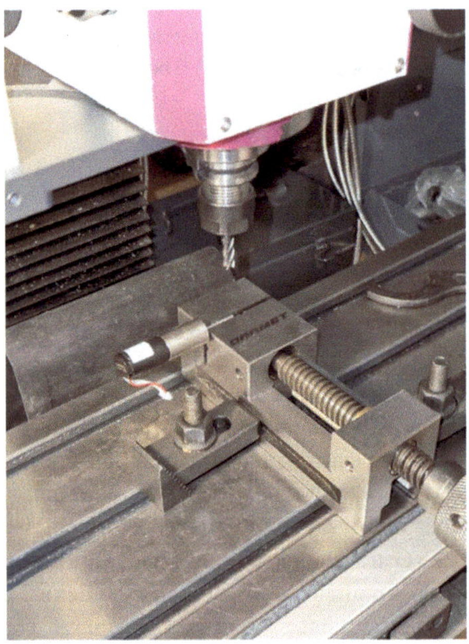

Fig. 7. Process planning for milling operations on the drive shaft [7].

Heavily loaded or high-precision components, such as shafts, bushings, gear housings, and load-transfer points, were manufactured from aluminum and steel using machining methods (shown in Fig. 7). The metal–PETG joints were achieved without complications, and the resulting mechanical stability confirmed that this hybrid approach is an appropriate pathway for prostheses intended for adolescent users, who generate higher loads than younger children.

The integration of the hand and wrist drives within the PETG forearm structure demonstrated that a hybrid design—comprising a printed load-bearing framework and metallic force-transmitting components—can be realized in an economical yet durable manner. In doing so, one of the most frequently reported barriers in the literature was addressed, namely the lack of space for multifunctional drive systems in pediatric prostheses.

3.2 Finishing Processing and Final Assembly

After printing all PETG components, they were subjected to careful finishing processing (shown in Fig. 8), which included the removal of supports, smoothing of contact areas, and adjustment of cooperating surfaces. PETG, owing to its higher elasticity compared to brittle materials, made it possible to achieve smooth surfaces in the mounting zones without the risk of chipping or micro-cracking typically observed with PLA.

Detailed fitting of bushings, shafts, and bearings was performed in the regions where mechanical components interact, allowing for smooth motion without vibrations or stepwise transitions. PETG, being more resistant to abrasion, provided improved operating conditions for moving elements, especially in areas with limited space for additional reinforcements.

The inner surface of the socket was prepared with equal care, with the PETG material enabling the required smoothness for contact with soft tissues. At the site of the FSR sensor installation, the stiffness of the substrate was made uniform to ensure even pressure distribution and repeatable signal output. This stage was crucial for the correct functioning of the control system, as even minor differences in material deformation could affect the sensor's sensitivity.

The integration of electronics, wiring, the microcontroller, and the motor driver module proceeded without issues, and the PETG structure allowed stable mounting of components without the need for additional reinforcement. The final assembly demonstrated high precision of fit, proper cable routing, and no need for post-production adjustments. Once assembled, the prosthesis maintained low weight, high rigidity, and an aesthetically pleasing appearance, which is particularly important for devices intended for young users.

3.3 Evaluation of the Manufactured Prototypes

The evaluation of the manufactured prototypes was carried out through a multi-stage assessment combining virtual verification, analysis of the fabricated components, and functional testing of the assembled prosthesis. The virtual environment evaluation consisted of three interconnected steps. First, collision detection was performed in Autodesk Inventor using a fully constrained assembly model with all contact definitions enabled. The software's solid-interference detection and minimum-distance tracking functions were activated, allowing the identification of areas with the smallest technological clearances and potential points of mechanical interference. Although the collision-checking tool also registers intersections with hidden bodies—which limits the precision of

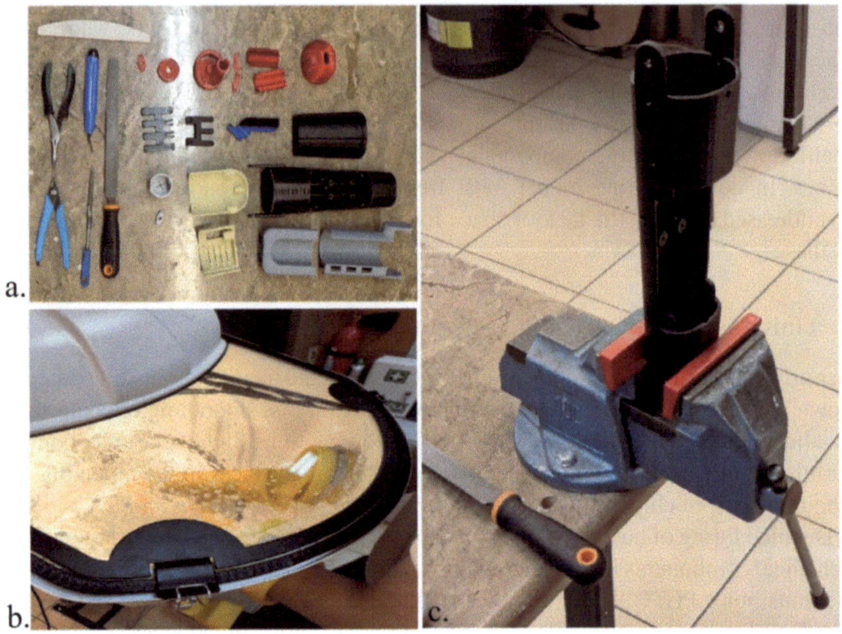

Fig. 8. a. – tools used in finishing processes, together with one of the first prototypes of the designed prosthesis (on the right) b. – finishing process of products obtained using Polyjet technology c. – workstation for finishing operations [7].

the analysis—the results nonetheless enabled targeted correction of specific housing geometries and cable-routing channels.

In the second step, the ranges of motion of the prosthetic joints were determined by defining kinematic pairs and constraints corresponding to the real device's mechanical limits. Extreme positions of the hand mechanism and wrist rotation module were recorded to verify that the intended functional workspace of the prosthesis was achievable without obstruction. The third part of the virtual evaluation focused on verifying the shape-based fitting of the prosthetic socket to the residual limb. Using triangular meshes obtained from 3D scanning, the socket model and limb model were aligned within a shared coordinate system in Meshmixer. As shown in Fig. 9, the fitting was assessed by positioning the socket over the reference surface of the residual limb, generating longitudinal and transverse control cross-sections, and inspecting areas of close contact. Variants including soft-liner thickness were also tested by applying positive surface offsets to the limb mesh. This analysis made it possible to identify regions requiring local shape corrections, particularly in zones susceptible to increased surface pressure, and to verify the continuity of contact and the presence of required ventilation clearances. This form of shape-matching evaluation ensured anatomical accuracy without the need for numerical deviation-map computation.

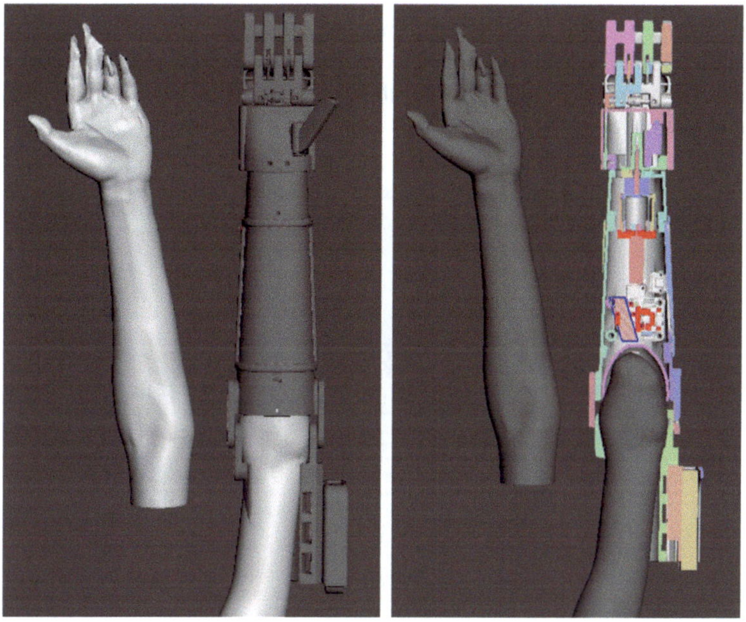

Fig. 9. Analysis of Residual Limb Fitting and Comparison with the Healthy Limb [7].

The evaluation of the physical prototypes confirmed that the geometric assumptions adopted during CAD modelling were successfully transferred into the manufactured components. All interfaces between the socket, forearm, and mechatronic modules aligned precisely with the digital model, demonstrating that the integration of the AutoMedPrint base geometry with custom mechanical assemblies was correct. The dimensional consistency of PETG-printed components was particularly important, as it ensured that the internal mounting spaces for motors, drives, and electronics required no post-production adjustments.

The manufacturing process further validated the design decisions. Components produced via FFF exhibited stable geometry and high-quality surfaces, enabling seamless integration with machined aluminum and steel elements such as shafts, bushings, and load-bearing contact points. This hybrid construction approach proved effective for creating mechanisms capable of withstanding operational loads typical for adolescent users. The functional evaluation, documented in the corresponding figures, demonstrated that the prosthesis is capable of performing essential daily-life tasks with stability, precision, and controlled movement. In the first series of tests, the prosthesis successfully lifted a 1 kg bag, confirming that the hand drive provides sufficient gripping force for handling relatively heavy objects. Holding a pen further demonstrated the device's ability to execute precise, low-force grasps—one of the most challenging tasks for compact mechatronic mechanisms.

In subsequent tests, the prosthesis held a book and a cup without slippage, benefiting from both the gripping mechanism and the active wrist rotation module. These tasks highlighted the importance of wrist positioning for natural object manipulation. The prosthesis also performed a cabinet-opening task, requiring simultaneous gripping and torque application. The self-locking wrist mechanism maintained positional stability throughout the movement, underscoring the ergonomic and mechanical suitability of the design [7].

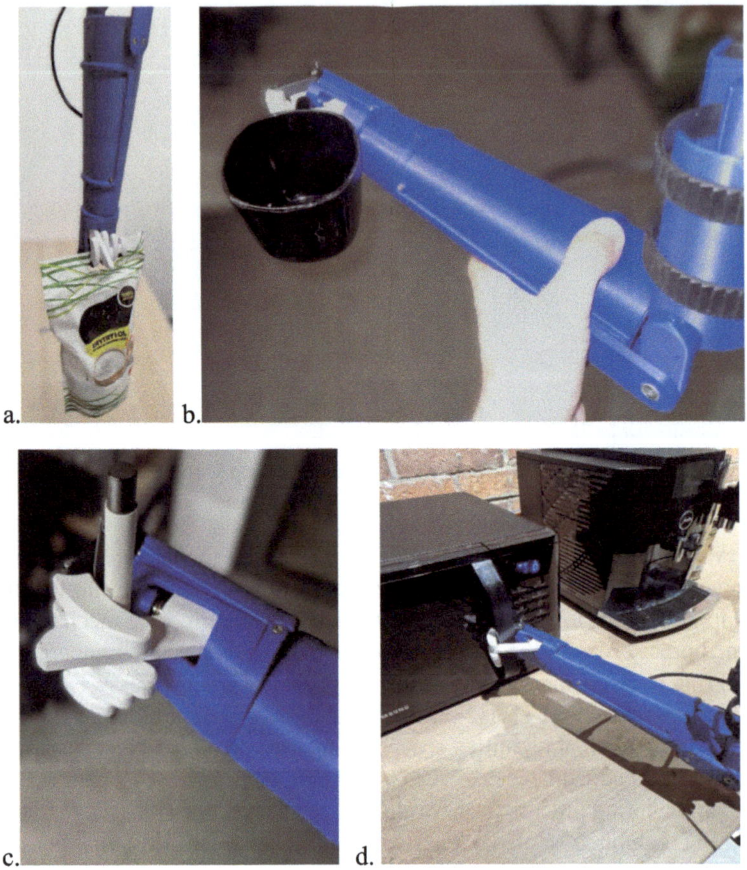

Fig. 10. Presentation of functional tests: a – holding a sugar packet, b – holding a cup, c – holding a pen, d – opening a microwave oven [7].

The functional evaluation of the physical prototype is presented in Fig. 10, illustrating representative daily-life tasks performed using the developed prosthesis [7]. Although the performed tests confirm functional feasibility, some of the obtained results remain qualitative in nature and should be interpreted with appropriate caution.

4 Discussion

The prototype presented in this article operated reliably and fulfilled the main design assumptions. However, since it has not yet been tested by the intended end user, its real-world performance cannot be fully verified. During the final development phase, several aspects were identified that may need improvement before clinical implementation, including socket fit and user-control mechanisms. These limitations largely result from the absence of direct patient participation during evaluation [7].

Nevertheless, the tests performed so far show promising results and confirm that such a low-cost solution is feasible. The use of the AutoMedPrint system significantly shortened the design workflow, while the chosen manufacturing methods enabled rapid iteration and yielded components with strength adequate for everyday use. To comprehensively confirm the device's safety and functionality, additional studies — particularly destructive testing — are required to establish safe operating limits and ensure long-term durability [7]. It must be clearly emphasized that the prototype has not yet undergone clinical testing with the intended end user. Therefore, its real-world functional performance, long-term comfort, and usability cannot be fully validated at this stage. This limitation should be addressed in future work through controlled clinical trials and extended user-based evaluations.

5 Conclusions

This work presents a prototype of a low-cost, anatomically individualized mechatronic upper-limb prosthesis for a juvenile patient with congenital transradial amputation. The design was based on the AutoMedPrint module, which served as the foundation for integration with mechanical, electronic, and drive components. The prosthesis was equipped with two independent mechanisms—a hand-grasping unit and a 90° wrist rotation module—controlled by an Arduino Nano microcontroller and an FSR pressure sensor. Structural elements were manufactured using additive technologies with polymer materials, complemented by machining for components requiring higher strength.

Functional testing confirmed the ability to perform basic daily activities, such as grasping objects, manipulating a door handle, and lifting items up to 1 kg, while maintaining a total mass (0.89 kg) comparable to that of a natural limb. The results highlight the practical potential of AutoMedPrint and additive manufacturing in the development of affordable, anatomically tailored prostheses, while also indicating the need for further clinical and ergonomic validation, durability testing, and long-term usability assessment.

Acknowledgments. This research was funded by the grant 0612/SBAD/3642, Funded by the Ministry of Science and Higher Education, Poland. Part of the studies were realized in scope of the grant entitled "Biomedical Innovations through Digital Transformation of Additive Technologies and Knowledge Exchange – BIOMEDIX" supported by ERASMUS+ (2024-1-LV01-KA220-HED-000255929).

References

1. Enderle J, Blanchard S, Bronzino J (2012) Introduction to biomedical engineering. Elsevier Academic Press, Amsterdam
2. Dolatkowski M, Stróżyk J (2024) Projektowanie wytwarzanych przyrostowo protez kończyny górnej dla przypadku amputacji obustronnej. Praca Dyplomowa. Politechnika Poznańska, Poznań

3. Biddiss EA, Chau TT (2007) Upper limb prosthesis use and abandonment: a survey of the last 25 years. Prosthetics Orthot Int 31(3):236–257
4. Sjöberg L, Lindner H, Hermansson L (2018) Long-term results of early myoelectric prosthesis fittings: a prospective case–control study. Prosthetics Orthot Int 42(5):527–533
5. Egermann M, Kasten P, Thomsen M (2009) Myoelectric hand prostheses in very young children. Int Orthop 33(4):1101–1105
6. Postema K, Rijke RA, van Limbeek J, van der Donk V, Poelma MJ (1999) Prosthesis rejection in children with a unilateral congenital arm defect. Clin Rehabil 13(3):243–249
7. Dolatkowski M (2025) Design and testing of a low-cost. In: Anatomically customized mechatronic hand prosthesis. Praca Dyplomowa. Politechnika Poznańska, Poznań
8. Górski F (2025) Computer aided design of 3D printable anatomically shaped medical devices: methodologies and applications. CRC Press, Taylor & Francis, Boca Raton
9. Górski F et al (2025) Automation of design of modular upper limb prostheses. In: Facta Universitatis, Series: Mechanical Engineering. University of Nis, Serbia
10. Górski F et al (2024) Individualized 3D printed orthopaedic and prosthetic devices using AutoMedPrint technology – methodologies and examples. Adv. Sci. Technol. Res. J. 18(6):145–158
11. Ottobock: Product Information 8E70-61081. Ottobock Official Website. Available at: https://www.ottobock.com/en-ex/product/8E70-61081 (Accessed 9 Aug 2025)
12. Aether Biomedical: Zeus hand – product information. Aether Biomedical Official Website Available at: https://www.aetherbiomedical.com/zeus-hand#zeusFeatures. Accessed 9 Aug 2025
13. Hy5: Hy5 Prosthetic Hand – Product Brochure. Hy5 Official Document. Available at: https://static1.squarespace.com/static/5a7c1da98dd041a5e11ca255/t/5ced2b355345 0aa6bd467d16/1559046970554/Hy5_Brochure_web.pdf. Accessed 9 Aug 2025
14. Fillauer: Jaws – Prosthetic Terminal Device. Fillauer Official Website. Available at: https://fillauer.com/product/jaws/. Accessed 9 Aug 2025
15. Górski F, Zawadzki P, Wichniarek R, Kuczko W, Słupińska S, Żukowska M (2022) Automated design and rapid manufacturing of low-cost customized upper limb prostheses. J. Phys.: Conf. Ser. 2198(1):012040

Advanced Materials, Characterization, and Performance Validation in Medical Additive Manufacturing

Study of Thermal and Mechanical Properties of Additively Manufactured PLA in the Context of Hand Orthosis Design

Aleksandra Grohs[1](✉), Filip Górski[1], Magdalena Żukowska[1], Wiesław Kuczko[1], Przemysław Zawadzki[1], Błażej Gabryszewski[1], Sabina Siwiec-Troszczyńska[2], and Radosław Wichniarek[1]

[1] Poznan University of Technology, Faculty of Mechanical Engineering, Piotrowo 3, 60-965 Poznań, Poland
aleksandra.grohs@doctorate.put.poznan.pl
[2] Poznan University of Medical Sciences, Fredry 10, 61-701 Poznan, Poland

Abstract. This study evaluates the thermal stability, mechanical performance, and geometric accuracy of polylactic acid (PLA) manufactured using fused deposition modeling (FDM) in the context of orthosis design. PLA is widely used in medical 3D printing due to its accessibility, biocompatibility, and ease of processing; however, its anisotropy, surface roughness, and low softening temperature impose functional constraints in orthotic applications. A hand orthosis model was produced in both vertical and horizontal print orientations, assessed for dimensional accuracy, subjected to three-point bending tests including cyclic loading, and monitored using thermal imaging during printing. Findings indicate that vertical orientation provides superior surface quality and higher bending stiffness, while geometric deviations remained within clinically acceptable limits. Thermal imaging showed stable printing conditions, and mechanical testing demonstrated that PLA withstands forces exceeding those typically generated by spastic or contractured muscles. The results suggest that PLA is suitable for short-term or pediatric orthoses, though limitations such as brittleness and thermal sensitivity should be considered. Future work should explore alternative lattice geometries, connection methods, and comparisons with higher-performance polymers.

Keywords: PLA · 3D printing · Orthoses · FDM · Material properties

1 Introduction

In recent years, 3D printing has become one of the most influential technologies enabling personalized medical solutions. It is used to fabricate anatomical models, assist in surgical planning [1], and manufacture customized rehabilitation and orthotic devices [2, 3]. In orthotics, 3D printing accelerates the design and production process by allowing accurate reproduction of patient anatomy and creating geometries that cannot be achieved through traditional fabrication methods [4, 5].

F. Górski et al. (Eds.): MANUFACTURING 2026, LNME, pp. 143–157, 2026.
https://doi.org/10.1007/978-3-032-23089-8_12

Numerous studies indicate that 3D-printed orthoses can offer clinical effectiveness and user comfort comparable to conventional devices, while also reducing production time and enabling easy design modifications [6]. This is particularly important in pediatric orthotics, where frequent size changes increase cost and material consumption [7]. The ability to locally adjust stiffness, perforation patterns, and wall thickness makes additive manufacturing a promising direction in modern orthotics, enabling lightweight, functional, and patient-specific devices [8, 9].

Material selection directly affects the effectiveness, comfort, and safety of an orthosis. One of the key considerations is the skin's sensitivity to localized pressure. Sustained pressure above approximately 32 mmHg can impair perfusion and lead to irritation or skin damage, while much lower pressures may already be perceived as discomfort [10]. The thresholds for perceiving pressure are significantly lower, so even minor localised misalignments can be felt by the user as discomfort [11]. Therefore, dimensional accuracy is crucial – small geometric deviations may produce local pressure peaks which affect user comfort and safety [12].

Thermal and moisture comfort is equally important. Heat and sweat accumulation can cause maceration or irritation; thus, materials with adequate vapor permeability and appropriately designed perforation improve skin condition [13]. Biocompatibility is essential, especially for children and individuals with a tendency to put their hands in the mouth. While PLA is generally biocompatible, additives or colorants may cause irritation [14]. For patients with spasticity or contractures, the material must also withstand forces generated by muscles and tendons. Clinical studies indicate that deforming forces in the hand can reach several tens of newtons, requiring sufficient stiffness and safety margin from the orthotic material [15, 16]. Overall, orthotic materials must ensure even pressure distribution, ventilation, biocompatibility, resistance to spastic forces, and the ability to maintain shape under daily use.

PLA is a popular FDM material due to its biodegradability, low mass, ease of printing, and minimal warping. It requires relatively low extrusion temperatures and produces dimensionally stable prints. However, in the case of PLA processed through FDM, surface exhibits visible layer lines and micro-roughness, which may increase friction against the skin [17].

Extruded PLA exhibits strong anisotropy: mechanical performance depends heavily on print orientation and infill pattern [18]. Inappropriate orientation can significantly reduce strength under bending or torsion. Its low glass-transition temperature (50–60 °C) increases the risk of deformation in hot environments or direct sunlight. PLA has low thermal conductivity (~0.16 W/m·K), which reduces heat transfer to the skin but also risks local heat accumulation if ventilation is insufficient [19]. Due to micro-porosity typical of FDM, moisture retention and bacterial accumulation are possible, although antimicrobial PLA variants are being developed [20]. Despite these limitations, PLA remains an appealing material for short-term, pediatric, or educational orthoses due to its printability, availability, and low cost.

2 Motivation and Aim for the Study

Evaluating PLA properties is essential because orthotic effectiveness depends directly on thermal stability, mechanical strength, and geometric accuracy. PLA must resist forces generated by spastic or contracted muscles, maintain precise anatomical fit, and remain dimensionally stable near body temperature. Moreover, small dimensional inaccuracies (0.5–1 mm) can meaningfully affect comfort and function.

Given these requirements and PLA's known limitations, a systematic assessment is required to verify its suitability for orthotic applications.

The aim of this work is to evaluate the thermal, mechanical, and geometric properties of PLA in the context of orthosis design, with particular attention to shape stability, resistance to therapeutic loads, and dimensional accuracy of patient-specific components. Previous studies by the team have shown that it's viable to use it for the traumatic hand orthoses [21], while not really good for ankle foot orthoses. Overview of the research plan is shown in the Fig. 1.

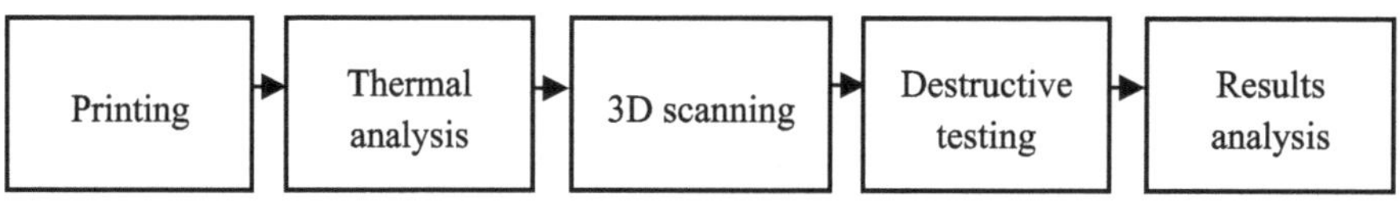

Fig. 1. Research overview

3 Materials and Methods

3.1 Material

A patient-specific hand orthosis model generated with the AutoMedPrint [22] system was used (Fig. 2) PLA filament (1.75 mm) in grey color provided by Fiberlogy served as the printing material.

3.2 Printing Parameters

Models were printed using a Bambu Lab P1S FDM printer with a 0.4-mm nozzle. Printing parameters followed the default "Generic PLA" profile. Key settings included in the Table 1. Photos of model are shown in the Fig. 3.

The models printed in the vertical configuration were manufactured in sequence, with the upper part completed in 01 h 59 min 30 s and the lower part in 02 h 10 min 01 s. In comparison, the models printed in the horizontal configuration required 01 h 59 min 37 s for the upper part and 02 h 25 min 00 s for the lower part. In total, five samples were printed in each orientation, then cleaned of supports using pliers and subsequently weighed. After preparation, all models were stored in plastic bags placed inside a semi-transparent container and kept in a shaded location.

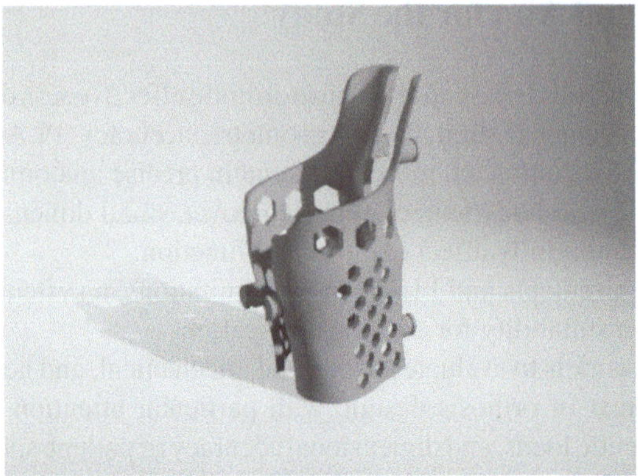

Fig. 2. Model of orthosis

Table 1. Key printing parameters

Parameter	Value	Parameter	Value
Nozzle temp.	220 °C	Layer height	0,20 mm
Table temp.	45 °C	Track width	0,42/0,45 mm
Cooling	100%	Filling	15, 00%
Velocity (ext. wall)	60 mm/s	No of outlines	3
Type of support	tree	Threshold angle	20 ° (ver)/ 25 ° (hor)

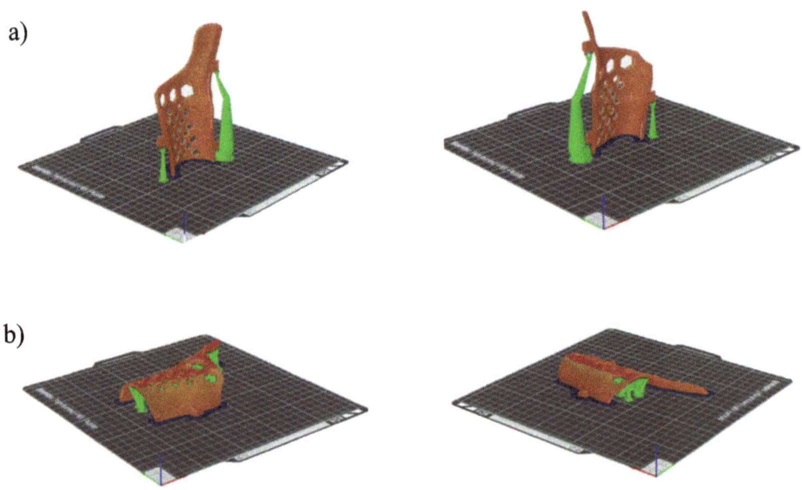

Fig. 3. Printed models a) vertical print configuration b) horizontal print configuration

3.3 Methods of Testing

Mechanical Testing. Three-point bending tests were conducted using a SUNPOC WDW-5D-HS universal testing machine. Custom printed supports were mounted on the fixture. Each model was placed on the support pins, secured with coated wire, and loaded via the testing head (Fig. 4).

Two test types were performed:

Cyclic (fatigue) loading: 20 cycles at 20–100 N and 20 cycles at 20–200 N.
Strength testing: Samples were loaded to failure

Measured parameters included maximum force (F_m), breaking force (FB), displacement (d), and the FB/F_m ratio indicating fracture abruptness – see formula (1).

$$FB/F_m \tag{1}$$

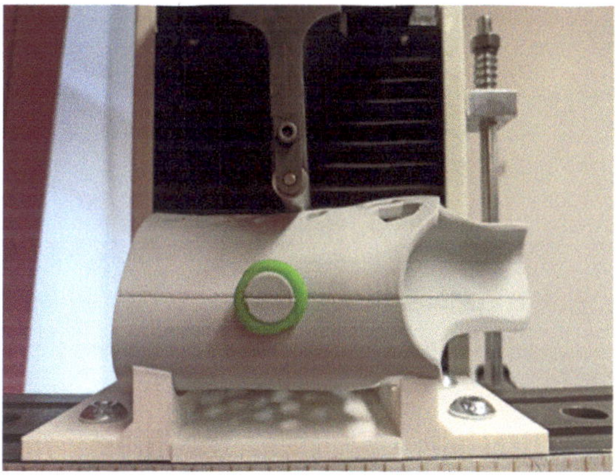

Fig. 4. Three-point bending station

Thermal Imaging. Thermal behavior during printing was recorded using a FLIR T530 infrared camera (320 × 240 px, 3 fps) positioned 80 cm from the printer. Three recording sessions were analyzed in FLIR Research Studio. Key temperature metrics included nozzle and bed stability, surface temperatures shortly after deposition, and temperature distribution across central and lateral regions. Thermal imaging camera station is presented in Fig. 5.

Based on the data obtained six characteristic thermal parameters were compared, describing: the stability of the work table temperature (*Linia 2*), the stability of the nozzle temperature (*Linia 1*), the temperatures of points shortly after printing (*Kwadrat 1* and *Kwadrat 2*), the temperature of the central areas (*Kwadrat 3* and *Kwadrat 4*). The measurement report is shown in Fig. 6.

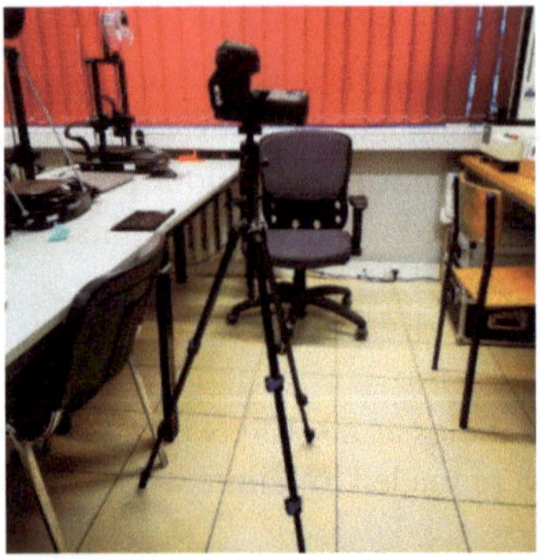

Fig. 5. Thermal imaging camera station

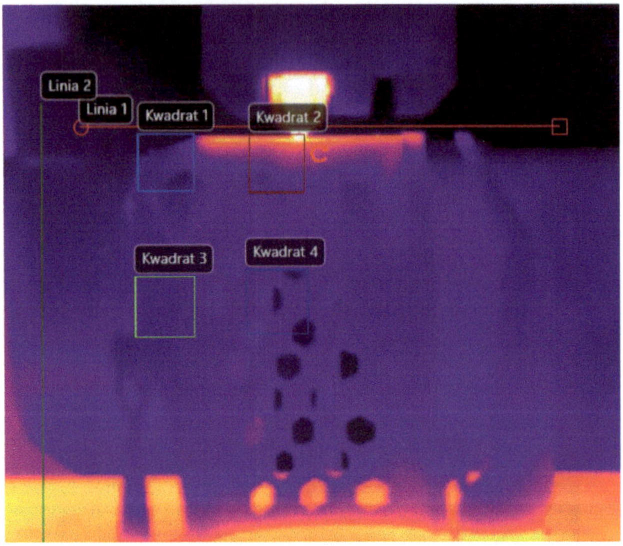

Fig. 6. Thermal imaging measurement report

Geometric Analysis. Printed models were scanned using an EinScan Pro 2X 2020 scanner. Point clouds were processed into STL geometry and compared against the nominal CAD model in GOM Inspect. The measuring station consisting of a scanner, a turntable and a computer is visible in the Fig. 7.

Six reference measurement points were analyzed for each orthosis half. The Fig. 8 shows the measurement points for deviations in the upper and lower parts of the orthosis.

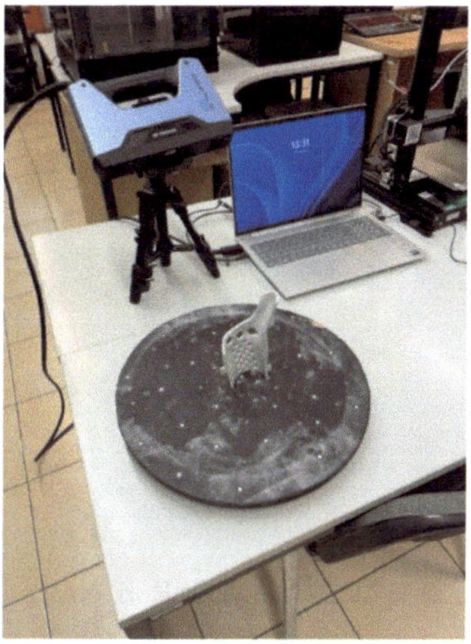

Fig. 7. The measuring station

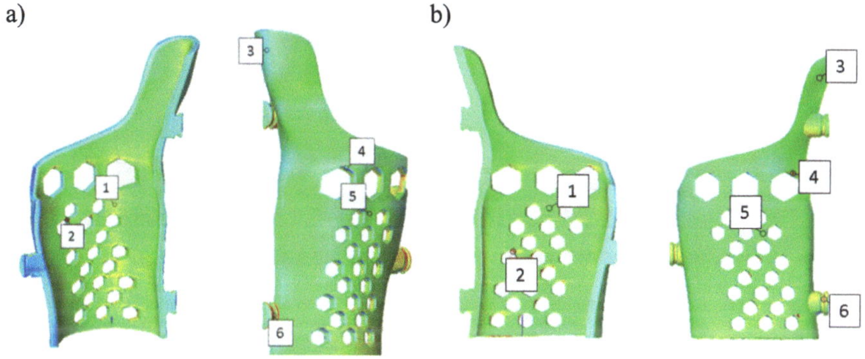

Fig. 8. a) Measurement points on the lower part of the orthosis, b) Measurement points on the upper part of the orthosis

4 Results

4.1 Geometric Properties

Ten orthoses were printed; two required reprinting due to nozzle clogging. Sample printouts are shown in the Fig. 9.

Observed print artefacts included first-layer expansion, stringing, staircase effect, and support scarring (Fig. 10). Vertical prints showed fewer defects and smoother surfaces. Weight deviations averaged ~4–5% from slicing estimates. See Table 2 for reference.

Dimensional deviations remained mostly within ±0.4 mm. Larger deviations were observed in areas with abrupt cross-section changes or near support interfaces.

The results of the analysis of selected measuring points in the GOM inspect program are shown in the Table 3.

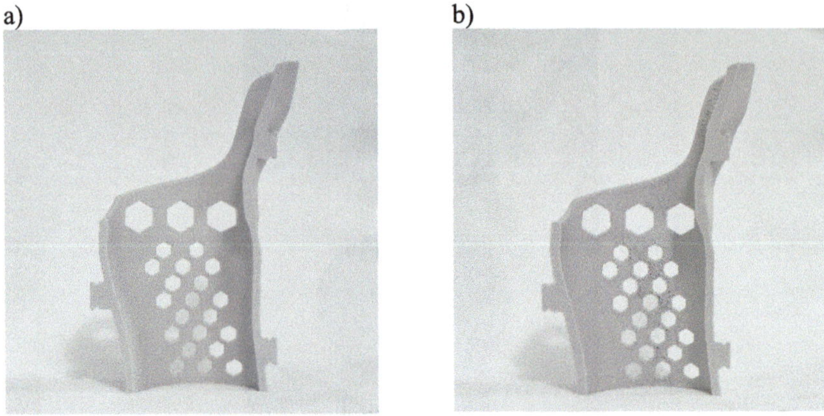

Fig. 9. a) Vertical printout b) Horizontal printout

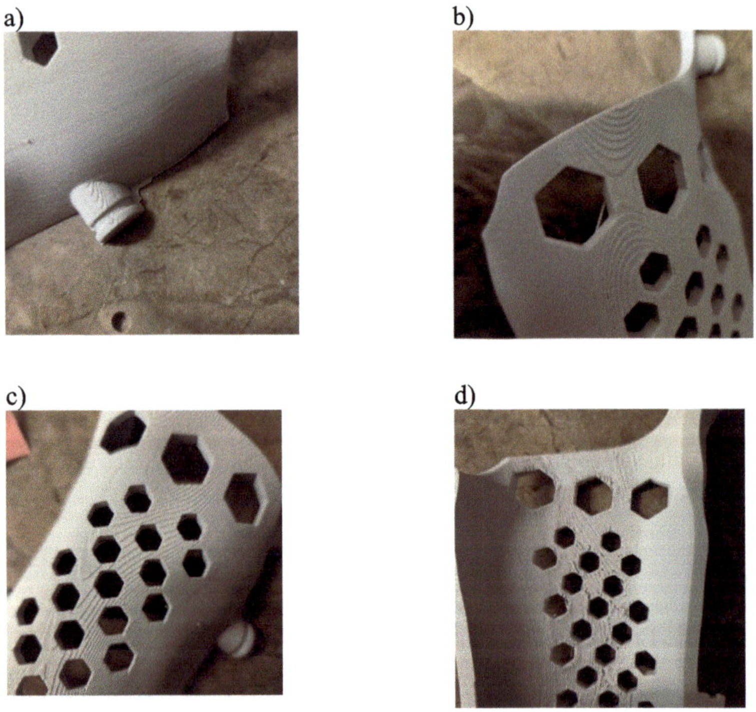

Fig. 10. Printing errors and surface distortions: a) first-layer expansion, b) stringing artifacts, c) staircase effect, d) support scarring

Table 2. Orthosis weight

Orientation	Upper/lower half	Estimated weight of used model material [g]	Mean weight [g]	Deviation [%]
Vertical	lower	36,7	35,1	4,5%
Vertical	upper	29,0	27,8	4,1%
Horizontal	lower	36,0	34,3	4,6%
Horizontal	upper	28,2	26,7	5,5%

Table 3. Results of orthosis scan measurements

Part	Point	Average [mm]	Min [mm]	Max [mm]	Dev [mm]
upper vertical	1	0,01	−0,03	0,05	0,03
	2	0,34	0,22	0,50	0,10
	3	−0,06	−0,20	0,04	0,10
	4	0,43	0,22	0,62	0,14
	5	−0,05	−0,10	0,01	0,04
	6	0,37	0,32	0,42	0,04
lower vertical	1	0,02	−0,02	0,13	0,05
	2	0,47	0,40	0,57	0,07
	3	−0,33	−0,60	−0,12	0,22
	4	−0,25	−0,33	−0,20	0,05
	5	−0,04	−0,06	−0,02	0,02
	6	0,42	0,39	0,45	0,02
upper horizontal	1	0,18	0,13	0,25	0,04
	2	0,83	0,64	1,30	0,24
	3	-0,07	-0,41	0,09	0,19
	4	0,14	-0,01	0,37	0,13
	5	-0,03	-0,11	0,05	0,05
	6	0,20	0,18	0,24	0,02
lower horizontal	1	0,14	0,06	0,27	0,08
	2	0,77	0,62	1,07	0,16
	3	-0,05	-0,18	0,05	0,08
	4	-0,04	-0,11	0,08	0,07
	5	-0,08	-0,12	-0,02	0,03
	6	0,38	0,32	0,45	0,05

4.2 Mechanical Properties

Vertical samples achieved higher bending stiffness ($F_m \approx 470$ N) than the horizontal ones (≈ 394 N). Breaking forces were comparable, though vertical samples exhibited more abrupt failure (lower FB/F_m ratio). Fatigue testing caused no damage at 100 N; initial degradation appeared at 200 N. See Table 4 and Figs. 11, 12 and 13 for reference.

Table 4. Mechanical testing results

Orientation	Sample no	F_m [N]	FB [N]	FB/ F_m [−]	d max [mm]
vertical	1	464,2	381,8	0,8	9,3
vertical	2	480,0	337,6	0,7	7,9
vertical	3	471,6	371,0	0,8	8,1
vertical	4	464,0	316,4	0,7	8,5
horizontal	2	371,0	368,6	1,0	8,7
horizontal	3	415,8	388,0	0,9	9,3
horizontal	4	385,4	343,8	0,9	8,9
horizontal	5	404,4	386,6	1,0	9,0
$\bar{X}$ vertical	–	470,00	351,7	0,8	8,4
$\bar{X}$ horizontal	–	394,2	371,8	0,9	9,0
σ vertical	–	6,6	26,2	0,1	0,6
σ horizontal	–	17,2	17,9	<0,1	0,2

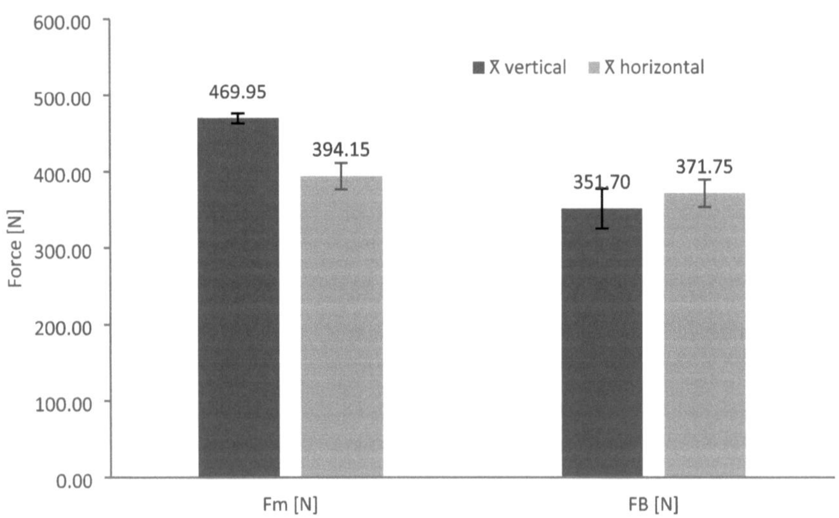

Fig. 11. Vertical and horizontal bending test results

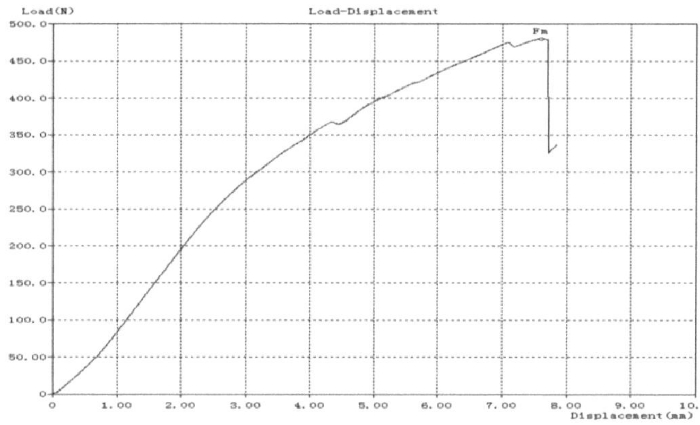

Fig. 12. Load-displacement of a vertically printed orthosis

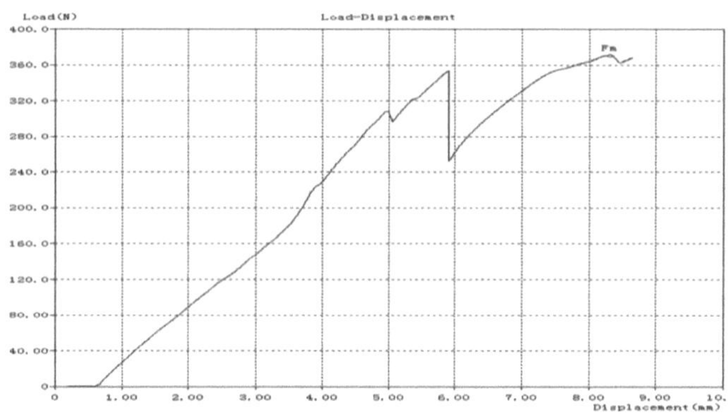

Fig. 13. Load-displacement of a horizontally printed orthosis

Fractures occurred primarily at support contact zones and regions of concentrated stress near the hexagonal lattice (Fig. 14). Samples tended to shift at the connection points during testing, influencing failure mode.

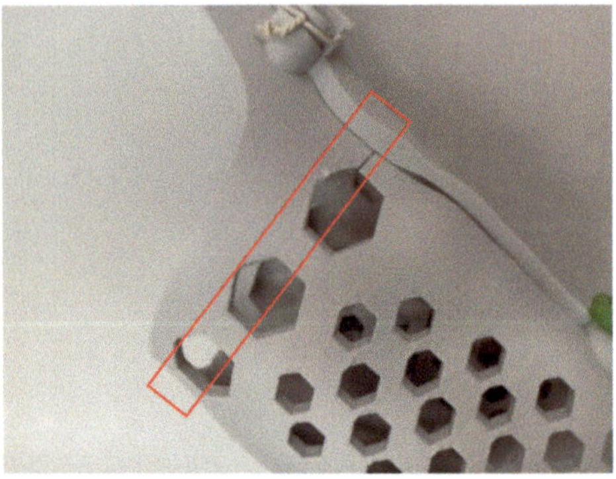

Fig. 14. Orthosis break

As a result of fatigue testing at an initial load of 100 N, no damage to the orthosis was observed. The effects of material degradation began to be noticeable only at a load of 200 N.

4.3 Thermal Analysis

Bed temperature remained stable (34.6–35.9 °C). Nozzle temperature fluctuated due to head motion but exhibited a consistent periodic pattern. Surface temperatures of freshly printed layers ranged from ~34 °C to 130 °C depending on proximity to the nozzle. Central regions retained heat longer than lateral zones. Due to the length of the process, Figs. 15 and 16 show excerpts from thermal imaging camera footage.

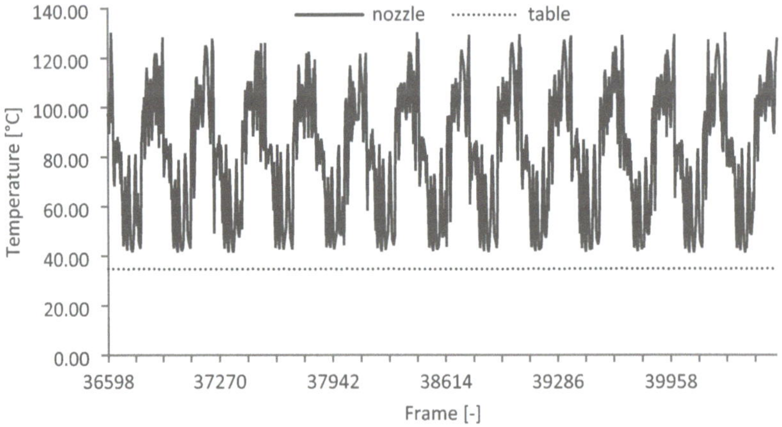

Fig. 15. Nozzle and table temperature graph

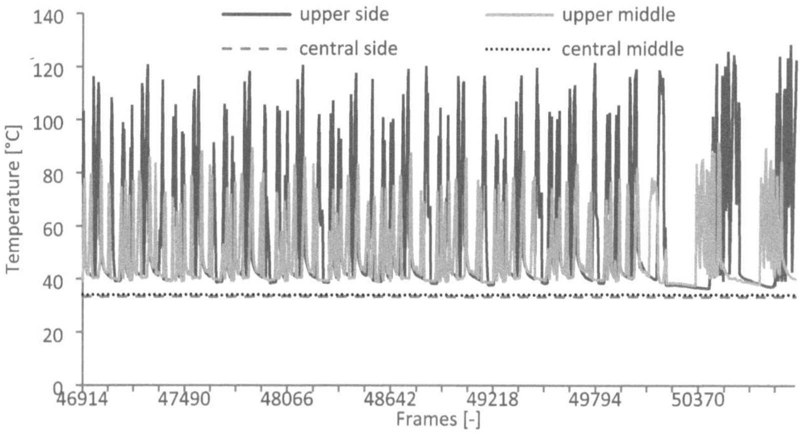

Fig. 16. Temperature graph of selected points during orthosis printing

5 Conclusions

The results of this study demonstrate that PLA, despite its known limitations, can serve as a suitable material for selected orthotic applications, particularly short-term devices and pediatric orthoses. The geometric accuracy achieved in both print orientations was clinically acceptable, with deviations generally below ±0.4 mm. Such discrepancies are unlikely to generate harmful local pressure peaks and can be further compensated using thin EVA padding.

Mechanical testing confirmed that PLA orthoses possess sufficient stiffness to counteract forces typically produced by spasticity or contractures, which rarely exceed several dozen newtons. Vertical prints offered significantly higher bending stiffness and superior surface quality, suggesting that this orientation should be preferred in orthotic production. Fracture patterns indicated no sharp splinters capable of injuring the patient, although the concentration of stresses around the hexagonal lattice highlights the need for re-evaluating perforation design. Alternative lattice structures such as Voronoi or gyroid could improve load distribution.

Thermal imaging demonstrated that printing conditions were stable and the material behaved predictably during deposition. Although PLA's relatively low softening temperature limits its use in hot environments, the temperatures relevant to daily orthosis wear do not pose a risk of deformation. Nevertheless, long-term exposure to sunlight remains a concern and warrants further investigation.

Overall, PLA's advantages – low mass, biocompatibility, affordability, and ease of printing – make it a practical choice for many orthotic applications. Its limitations, including brittleness and thermal sensitivity, suggest caution when designing devices subjected to significant dynamic loads or environmental stressors. Future work should include comparative testing with materials such as PCTG and nylon, evaluation of alternative connection mechanisms for multi-part orthoses, and optimization of lattice patterns to minimize stress concentrations.

Acknowledgements. The study was realized with support from Polish Ministry of Science and Education and Polish State Fund For Rehabilitation Of Disabled People (contract number BEA/000079/BF/D). Additional support was provided by the BIOMEDIX project, realized within the Erasmus+ programme.

References

1. Smolarek E, Górski F, Żukowska M, Słowik Ł, Okła M (2025) Partial maxillofacial reconstruction: design and additive manufacturing of individualized pre-and mid-surgery supplies. Adv. Sci. Technol. Res. J. 19(8):114–125. https://doi.org/10.12913/22998624/204756
2. Rengier F et al (2010) 3D printing based on imaging data: review of medical applications. Int J Comput Assist Radiol Surg 5(4):335–341. https://doi.org/10.1007/s11548-010-0476-x
3. Górski F (2025) Computer aided design of 3D printable anatomically shaped medical devices: methodologies and applications. CRC Press
4. Choo YJ, Boudier-Revéret M, Chang MC (2020) 3D printing technology applied to orthosis manufacturing: narrative review. Ann. Palliat. Med. 9(6):4262–4270. https://doi.org/10.21037/apm-20-1185
5. Gorski F et al (2025) Automation of design of modular upper limb prostheses. In: Facta Universitatis, Series mechanical engineering
6. Fang JJ, Lin CL, Tsai JY, Lin RM (2022) Clinical assessment of customized 3D-printed wrist orthoses. Appl Sci 12(22):11538. https://doi.org/10.3390/app122211538
7. Oud TAM, Lazzari E, Gijsbers HJH, Gobbo M, Nollet F, Brehm MA (2021) Effectiveness of 3D-printed orthoses for traumatic and chronic hand conditions: a scoping review. PLoS One 16(11):e0260271. https://doi.org/10.1371/journal.pone.0260271
8. Mavroidis C et al (2011) Patient specific ankle-foot orthoses using rapid prototyping. J Neuroeng Rehabil 8(1):1. https://doi.org/10.1186/1743-0003-8-1
9. Jańczak K, Górski F, Żukowska M, Rybarczyk JB, Barteczka T, Kuczko W (2025) The application of additive manufacturing technology in designing and producing individualized lower limb orthoses. Adv. Sci. Technol. Res. J. 19(7):346–359. https://doi.org/10.12913/22998624/204052
10. Lyder CH, Ayello EA (2008) Pressure ulcers: a patient safety issue. In: Patient safety and quality: an evidence-based handbook for nurses
11. Greenspan JD, McGillis SLB (1994) Thresholds for the perception of pressure, sharpness, and mechanically evoked cutaneous pain: effects of laterality and repeated testing. Somatosens Mot Res 11(4):311–317. https://doi.org/10.3109/08990229409028875
12. Atallah H, Qufabz T, Bakhsh HR, Ferriero G (2025) The current state of 3D-printed orthoses clinical outcomes: a systematic review. BMC Musculoskelet Disord 26(1):822. https://doi.org/10.1186/s12891-025-09070-4
13. Filingeri D, Havenith G (2015) Human skin wetness perception: psychophysical and neurophysiological bases. Temperature 2(1):86–104. https://doi.org/10.1080/23328940.2015.1008878
14. Castro JI et al (2022) Biocompatibility assessment of polylactic acid (PLA) and nanobioglass (n-BG) nanocomposites for biomedical applications. Molecules 27(11):3640. https://doi.org/10.3390/molecules27113640
15. Kawamura K et al (2022) Quantitative measurement of resistance force and subsequent attenuation during passive isokinetic extension of the wrist in patients with mild to moderate spasticity after stroke. J Neuroeng Rehabil 19(1):110. https://doi.org/10.1186/s12984-022-01087-3

16. Plantin J et al (2019) Quantitative assessment of hand spasticity after stroke: imaging correlates and impact on motor recovery. Front Neurol 10. https://doi.org/10.3389/fneur.2019.00836
17. Batista M, Del Sol I, Gómez-Parra Á, Vazquez-Martinez JM (2024) Tribological performance of additive manufactured PLA-based parts. Polymers 16(17):2529. https://doi.org/10.3390/polym16172529
18. Zohdi N, Yang R (2021) (Chunhui).: material anisotropy in additively manufactured polymers and polymer composites: a review. Polymers 13(19):3368. https://doi.org/10.3390/polym13193368
19. Blanco I, Cicala G, Recca G, Tosto C (2022) Specific heat capacity and thermal conductivity measurements of PLA-based 3D-printed parts with milled carbon fiber reinforcement. Entropy 24(5):654. https://doi.org/10.3390/e24050654
20. Brounstein Z, Yeager CM, Labouriau A (2021) Development of antimicrobial PLA composites for fused filament fabrication. Polymers 13(4):580. https://doi.org/10.3390/polym13040580
21. Górski F, Wichniarek R, Kuczko W, Żukowska M, Lulkiewicz M, Zawadzki P (2020) Experimental studies on 3D printing of automatically designed customized wrist-hand orthoses. Materials 13(18):4091. https://doi.org/10.3390/ma13184091
22. Górski F et al (2024) Individualized 3D printed Orthopaedic and prosthetic devices using AutoMedPrint technology – methodologies and examples. Adv. Sci. Technol. Res. J. 18(6):145–158. https://doi.org/10.12913/22998624/191548

DLP-Printed Titanium Nanocomposite Resin for Bioactive Interfacial Layers Promoting Bone Feeding and Healing at the Humerus–Plate Junction

Monica Rău[1], Răzvan Păcurar[1], Mircea Năsui[1], Augusta Oros[1], Eugen Guţiu[1], Marks Gorohovs[2], Jurijs Dehtjars[2], Elizabete Skrebele[2], Nikola Vitković[3], Dan Sorin Comsa[1], Ancuţa Păcurar[1], and Diana Elena Horincar[1](✉)

[1] Technical University of Cluj-Napoca, Cluj-Napoca, Romania
diana.horincar@campus.utcluj.ro
[2] Riga Technical University, Riga, Latvia
[3] University of Nis, Niš, Serbia

Abstract. Addressing the inherent limitations of conventional metallic implants —notably infection susceptibility and deficient long-term osseointegration, this study introduces a novel dual-performance platform for personalized orthopedic fixation. The geometry for the extra-articular distal humerus locking compression plate (LCP) was meticulously designed via CAD and fabricated using Digital Light Processing (DLP). The core innovation is the functionalized nanocomposite interfacial layer, which utilizes a photopolymer matrix exclusively reinforced with Titanium Dioxide (TiO_2) nanoparticles. This specific formulation is designed to potentially confer essential antimicrobial properties and significantly enhance long-term osseointegration, thereby transcending the constraints of current inert implants. Nanocomposite samples were subjected to rigorous characterization, including FTIR for structural analysis and PES for assessing surface chemistry and the elemental state of Ti. Concurrently, a Finite Element Analysis (FEA) model was developed and utilized to optimize stress and strain distributions under critical biomechanical loading conditions. This integrated methodological approach establishes a robust protocol for developing a new class of personalized orthopedic implants with optimized mechanical and biological performance.

Keywords: Bioactive Nanocomposite · Titanium Nanocomposite Resin · Additive Manufacturing · Digital Light Processing · Material Characterization

1 Introduction

The successful management of complex bone defects requires fixation devices that merge mechanical precision with robust biological functionality. Personalized Patient-Specific Implants (PPIs) fabricated via Additive Manufacturing (AM) have significantly

F. Górski et al. (Eds.): MANUFACTURING 2026, LNME, pp. 158–171, 2026.
https://doi.org/10.1007/978-3-032-23089-8_13

advanced geometric fit. However, despite the superior fit, the critical bone-implant interface remains highly vulnerable to failure due to infection and insufficient osseointegration. While Titanium (Ti) and its alloys are the established gold standard for their biocompatibility and long-term osseointegration [1], the recognized biological barriers necessitate a transition from passive Ti surfaces to actively functionalized nanocomposites. Traditional surface-coating strategies such as sol-gel films, plasma coatings, or hydrothermal surface functionalization provide localized bioactivity but are inherently limited by their weak mechanical anchorage to the metallic substrate. These thin layers are susceptible to delamination, cracking, and abrasive wear, especially under cyclic loading and micromotion at the bone–implant interface. Conversely, bulk nanocomposite approaches, in which nanoparticles are dispersed throughout the entire structural material, typically offer improved stability but may compromise global mechanical properties. High nanoparticle loadings can disrupt polymer cross-linking, reduce toughness, induce stress concentrations, and hinder the curing kinetics required for load-bearing applications [2].

Current state-of-the-art surface modification research focuses on AM-compatible nanocomposites, often relying on complex coatings [3–5]. Our approach integrates the functional material directly into the DLP photopolymer matrix, presenting a high-resolution manufacturing advantage. This study leverages Titanium Dioxide Nanoparticles (TiO_2) for their superior and demonstrated dual functionality: providing active antimicrobial control and promoting long-term osteogenesis by stimulating stem cell differentiation [6, 7]. This strategy circumvents the limitations of strictly osteoconductive or solely antibacterial materials. The DLP-printed TiO2 nanocomposite interface developed in this study represents an intermediary and hybrid strategy between these two extremes. Instead of forming a fragile surface coating or altering the entire bulk plate material, the photopolymer TiO2 nanocomposite is applied selectively as a dedicated interfacial layer only along the bone-contacting surface. This approach ensures stronger mechanical integration than conventional coatings due to layer-by-layer photopolymerization bonding. This positions the DLP-engineered nanocomposite as a stable, mechanically supported, and biologically active intermediary solution that leverages the advantages of both coatings and bulk composites while minimizing their respective limitations.

Although TiO2 nanoparticles are widely recognized for their osteoconductive and antimicrobial properties, their use also carries several limitations that must be acknowledged. Free or unbound TiO2 nanoparticles can generate reactive oxygen species (ROS) under UV or high-energy excitation, potentially leading to oxidative stress and dose-dependent cytotoxic effects on surrounding tissues. Additional concerns include bioavailability and systemic distribution, particularly the risk of nanoparticle release, accumulation in distant organs, or interference with cellular metabolic pathways. The biological behavior of TiO2 is also strongly influenced by its crystalline phase: anatase typically exhibits higher photocatalytic activity and ROS generation, while rutile presents greater chemical stability but reduced biological reactivity. However, despite these inherent safety advantages of matrix embedding, the authors acknowledge that comprehensive biological validation including cytotoxicity assays, inflammatory response evaluation, and long-term in vivo studies remains essential for fully establishing the clinical safety and performance of the TiO2 nanocomposite interface [8].

Considering these dual performance requirements, this research proposes a TiO_2-Nanocomposite Resin as an intermediary interface layer on the personalized plate. The primary objective is to rigorously characterize this dual-functional interface, validating the central hypothesis that this AM-compatible material and design protocol successfully transforms an inert fixation device into an active system.

2 Transition from Geometric Design to Bioactive Interface Development

2.1 CAD Methodology and Geometric Fidelity

The geometric model for the personalized fixation plate (PPI) for the extra-articular distal humerus was developed using the Method of Anatomical Features (MAF), integrated with the Characteristic Product Features (CPF) methodology [9, 10]. The process began with the acquisition of a pre-existing left humerus surface model from a 512x512 pixels CT scan 0.5 mm slice thickness) and was executed in CATIA V5. The core MAF involved utilizing spline curves and Subdivision Surfaces (SubD) to map the contact surface, which was refined by adding transversal curves based on surgeon recommendations. This advanced parametric approach guaranteed a precise conformity to the bone shape, evidenced by a high geometrical fidelity with a median deviation of approximately 0.1–0.2 mm. This superior fit successfully eliminates the need for intraoperative plate bending and optimizes pre-operative load transfer.

2.2 Titanium Nanocomposite for Bioactive Layer

Despite the superior mechanical fit achieved by the CAD model (Fig. 1), the implant-bone contact surface presents a critical biological bottleneck, requiring active osseointegration and antimicrobial protection. Addressing this challenge mandates a dedicated intermediary layer focused on three clinical aspects: infection control, enhanced osseointegration, and improved local structural stability. To meet these demands, we fabricated a Titanium Nanocomposite Resin. This composite is specifically engineered for dual functionality: the resin matrix, primarily featuring TiO_2, provides proven antimicrobial properties and promotes mesenchymal stem cell differentiation.

2.3 Nanocomposite Functionality

Concurrently, the incorporation of Titanium Nanoparticles (TiO_2) is designed to significantly enhance the layer's osteo-conductivity. These nanoparticles increase the active surface area, thereby promoting robust adhesion, proliferation, and differentiation of osteoblasts essential for rapid bone formation and stable implant integration. The TiO_2 colloidal precursor used in this study consisted of nanoparticles predominantly in the anatase crystalline phase, as specified by the supplier and confirmed by X-ray diffraction (XRD) peaks characteristic of anatase TiO_2 (Fig. 2). The selection of the anatase phase

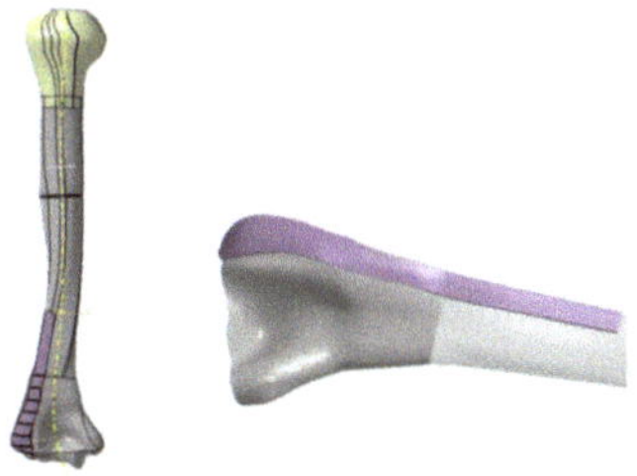

Fig. 1. Personalized 3D plate solid mod [11]

is intentional, as this polymorph exhibits well-documented bioactive behavior, including enhanced osteogenic stimulation, improved protein adsorption, and pronounced surface reactivity that supports early-stage osteoblast adhesion.

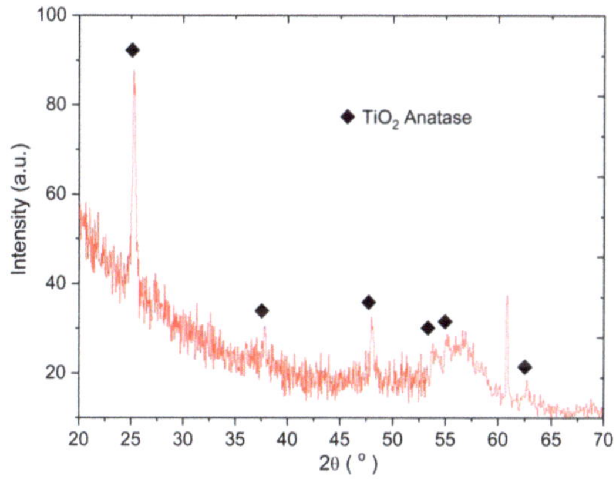

Fig. 2. XRD diffraction pattern of TiO2 nanoparticles

Ultimately, while the CAD model establishes the optimized mechanical geometry, the Titanium Nanocomposite Resin furnishes the necessary optimized biological functionality, effectively transforming the passive fixation device into an active system for bone regeneration support.

3 Materials and Methods

Following the successful parametric optimization of the plate's geometry via the CAD/MAF-CPF methodology (as detailed in Sect. 2), the subsequent phase focused rigorously on material engineering to functionalize the bone-implant interface. The customized fixation device requires a stable polymer matrix compatible with high-resolution Additive Manufacturing (SLA), but crucially, this matrix must be modified to ensure long-term clinical success. Specifically, the material must actively promote osseointegration and mitigate post-operative infection risk. Therefore, a critical step involved the meticulous synthesis and preparation of the novel Titanium Nanocomposite Resin. The following section outlines the precise protocol used to achieve homogeneous dispersion of the functional nanoparticles, ensuring the required rheological properties for 3D printing, and ultimately guaranteeing the superior biological functionality of the plate's contact surface.

The functionalization of the photopolymer matrix was achieved through the precise incorporation of TiO_2 colloidal nanoparticles into the Anycubic Water-Wash Resin+ HD Gray base (Fig. 3). The preparation protocol was meticulously executed in three distinct stages to ensure optimal filler dispersion and final print quality. In the first stage, gravimetric dosing of components, a TiO_2 colloidal solution dispersed in isopropyl alcohol was introduced into the base resin matrix at a proportion of 10 vol%. Corresponding to a nanoparticle concentration of 50 mmol. This concentration was selected based on preliminary studies aimed at balancing enhanced bioactive properties with acceptable rheological and curing stability. In the second stage, dispersion and deagglomeration, the TiO_2-resin mixture was subjected to ultrasonic processing for 10–15 min following initial mechanical blending. This sonication step was critical to achieve a homogeneous distribution of the TiO_2 nanoparticles and to minimize the formation of agglomerates within the polymer matrix, thereby ensuring uniform optical and mechanical properties throughout the printed parts. Finally, during the vacuum degassing stage, the composite mixture underwent a controlled vacuum process to remove entrapped air bubbles and residual solvent traces. This final step was essential to prevent the formation of voids or micro-porosities during the stereolithography printing process, ensuring high structural integrity and surface quality in the resulting 3D-printed components.

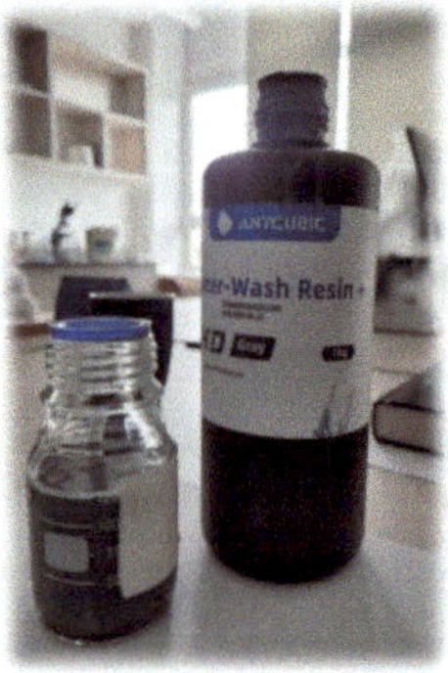

Fig. 3. Anycubic Water-Wash Resin + HD Gray - mixing of the resin with TiO_2 colloidal nanoparticles

4 Additive Manufacturing of Samples

The fabrication of the functionalized composite specimens was performed via Additive Manufacturing (AM), specifically employing Digital Light Processing (DLP) technology, which falls under the broader category of Stereolithography (SLA). This technique utilizes a digital light source to selectively cure liquid photopolymer resin layer-by-layer, a methodology selected for its proven capability in fabricating intricate geometries while delivering both excellent surface quality and high dimensional accuracy—attributes essential for medical implant prototypes [11].

The printing was conducted on an Anycubic Photon M3 Max DLP 3D printer. This specific equipment was chosen due to its large build volume and the precise control over exposure parameters it affords [12, 13].

A total of eight specimens (N = 8) were printed, each measuring 10 mm × 10 mm × 2 mm. All samples were oriented identically on the build platform to ensure reproducibility and minimize geometric variations attributable to anisotropic printing effects, thereby maintaining the homogeneity required for subsequent mechanical and biological testing (Fig. 4).

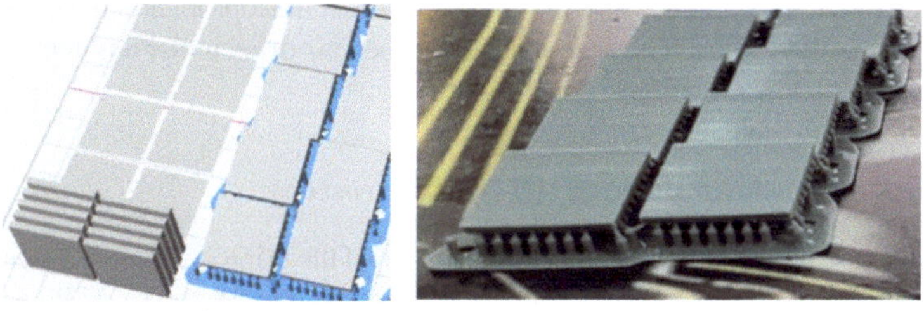

a) b)

Fig. 4. a) The samples prepared for printing b) Final printed samples before cleaning and post-curing

The primary printing parameters are summarized below: **technology**: Digital Light Processing (DLP); **equipment**: Anycubic Photon M3 Max; **layer thickness**: 0.05 mm; **normal exposure time**: 2.8 s; **slice parameter**: 0.05 mm; **material**: Water washable photopolymer resin mixed with TiO_2 nanoparticles; **support structures**: Small supports were added at the base and on floating areas for the samples.

The titanium nanocomposite resin was printed as a separate polymer sample. This printing batch required approximately 13 min, with a total resin consumption of 16.63 mL. Immediately following additive fabrication, the specimens underwent an essential post-processing protocol, consisting of washing to remove uncured resin residue and subsequent UV post-curing to achieve the maximal degree of polymer conversion.

The completion of these stabilization steps ensured the requisite structural integrity and surface homogeneity of the nanocomposite samples, thus preparing them for detailed experimental testing, analysis, and characterization.

5 Experimental Testing and Evaluation of Samples

5.1 Material Characterization

Understanding both the chemical composition and surface electronic properties of bioactive nanocomposite resins is essential for predicting and evaluating their possible performance at the bone-implant interface. The dynamic viscosity of the precursor solutions was measured using Brookfield Rheometer with a cone-plate geometry. The rheological characterization of composite solution in our case was made at shear rates in the range of 10 to 102 s^{-1}, which corresponds to medium shear viscosity (MSV). Chemical stability and functional group integrity influence molecular interactions with surrounding tissues, while surface potential characteristics can modulate protein adsorption and cellular adhesion. Therefore, the DLP-printed titanium nanocomposite resin samples were characterized using Fourier Transform Infrared (FTIR) spectroscopy to assess molecular structure and bonding, and Photoelectron Emission Spectroscopy (PEES) to evaluate surface energy states and determine electron work function values.

5.2 Sample Preparation

Prior to analysis, all samples were thoroughly washed in isopropanol and subsequently rinsed with distilled water. The specimens were then air-dried under ambient conditions before further characterization.

5.3 Fourier Transform Infrared (FTIR) Spectroscopy

The chemical structure and molecular composition of the printed composites were examined using a Bruker Tensor II spectrometer equipped with a Platinum ATR (Attenuated Total Reflectance) module. The spectra were collected in the wavenumber range of 4000–400 cm^{-1} with a spectral resolution of 4 cm^{-1}. Measurements were performed using OPUS software for both acquisition and data processing.

Before each measurement, a background spectrum was recorded under identical environmental conditions to eliminate atmospheric interference. The samples were placed in the center of the ATR crystal and pressed firmly against the diamond window to ensure optimal contact. Measurements were taken on different points of samples to verify the homogeneity of chemical composition of samples. The technique enabled the identification of characteristic vibrational modes of the polymer matrix and titanium-based nanofillers, serving as a molecular fingerprint of the composite material. Figure 5 shows the sample pressed against the diamond window.

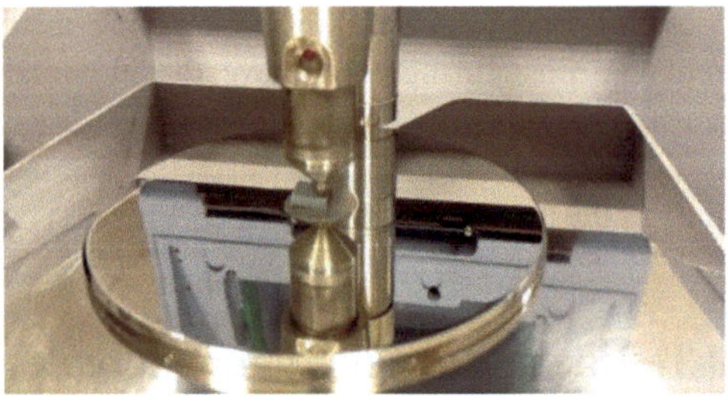

Fig. 5. DLP-printed titanium nanocomposite resin sample in FTIR spectrometer

5.4 Photoelectron Emission Spectroscopy (PEES)

Surface electronic properties were analyzed by photoelectron emission spectroscopy (PEES) using a custom-made photoelectron emission spectrometer, which can be seen in Fig. 6, operating under a high-vacuum environment of approximately 10^{-5} mmHg. A deuterium lamp served as a monochromatic ultraviolet source in the wavelength range of 200–277 nm (4.5–6.2 eV). The emitted photoelectrons were detected by a secondary electron multiplier, with an applied potential of 150 V at the cathode and 3 kV at the anode.

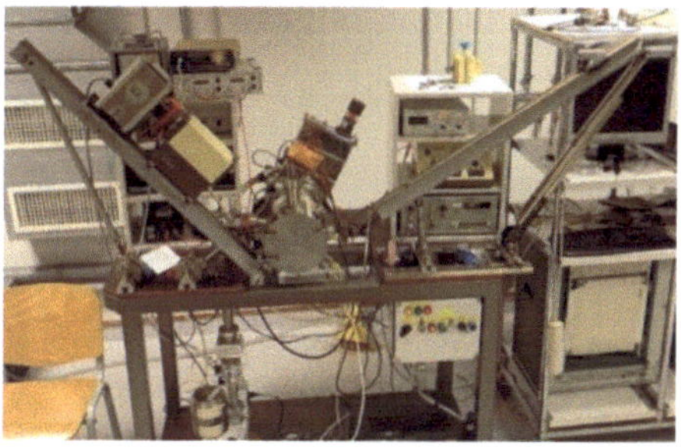

Fig. 6. Custom-made photoelectron emission spectrometer

The emitted electron count was recorded as a function of photon energy to obtain the photoemission yield curve. The electron work function (EWF) is the minimal amount of energy required to eject an electron from the surface of solid material. It was calculated from the intersection point of the linearized function Y/(dY/dhν) versus photon energy hν, according to Formula 1:

$$\frac{\mathrm{F}}{d\mathrm{F}/dhvv} = \frac{1}{\mathrm{m}}(hvv - \varphi_{\mathrm{m}}) \quad (1)$$

Y is the quantum yield, hν is a photon energy, φ is electron work function and m is a material-dependent constant.

The obtained electron work function values characterize the surface electronic potential and may indicate charge states favorable for bioactive interactions.

5.5 Results

The viscosity of the Anycubic Water-Wash Resin+ HD Gray base was evaluated before and after incorporation of the TiO_2 colloidal precursor solution to assess its effect on rheological properties. Measurements were performed using a rotational viscometer at 25 °C under controlled shear conditions. The base resin exhibited Newtonian behavior with a viscosity of approximately 850–900 mPa·s, consistent with the expected flow properties for stereolithography printing. After the addition of the TiO_2 colloidal solution (10 vol%, 50 mmol/L) and subsequent ultrasonic homogenization, the viscosity of the composite resin decreased to approximately 700–750 mPa·s. This reduction is attributed to the isopropyl alcohol medium in the colloidal solution, which acts as a diluent and improves flowability. Despite the decrease, the resin maintained sufficient rheological properties compatible with high-resolution 3D printing, confirming that the TiO_2 precursor was successfully incorporated without compromising processability.

The FTIR spectra of 8 samples showed nearly identical spectral profiles, with no observable blue or red shifts in the main peaks, indicating high chemical uniformity and reproducibility of the material. Only minor variations in band intensity were observed, which likely reflect slight differences in local nanoparticle distribution or surface roughness rather than compositional changes. Figure 7 shows the average FTIR spectra of DLP-printed titanium nanocomposite resin:

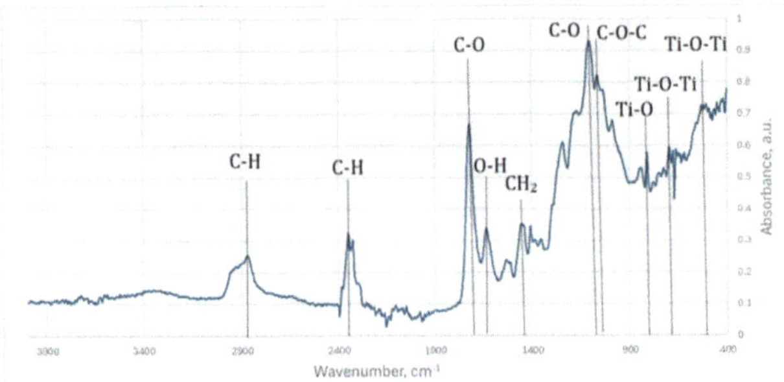

Fig. 7. FTIR spectra of DLP-printed titanium nanocomposite resin

FTIR spectra shows distinct peaks of methacrylate photopolymer resins: aliphatic C–H stretching at around 2860 and 2350 cm^{-1}, a strong ester C=O stretching band at 1721 cm^{-1}, CH2 bending at around 1450 cm^{-1}, and C–O–C stretching around 1060 cm^{-1} [14]. The most intense peak near 1100 cm^{-1} is typical for ester/ether C–O stretching. Bands at 805, 690 and 500 cm^{-1} are associated to the Ti-O and Ti-O-Ti, verifying the presence of titanium oxide species within samples [15–17].

PEES revealed EWF values for the eight tested DLP-printed titanium nanocomposite resin samples ranging from 4.51 to 4.59 eV (Fig. 8). The results demonstrated a high degree of reproducibility, with standard deviations between 0.004 and 0.023 eV, indicating stable surface electronic properties across identically fabricated specimens. Statistical analysis (t-test, 95% confidence) showed that samples 1–5 formed a statistically homogeneous group within the measurement error, whereas samples 7 and 8 exhibited slightly elevated work function values (4.58 ± 0.01 eV), differing significantly from the first group (4.53 ± 0.03 eV). Sample 6 (4.55 ± 0.02 eV) overlapped both distributions, suggesting possible localized surface differences or minor inconsistencies during printing or post-processing.

The overall narrow range of work function values confirms the good uniformity and repeatability of the photopolymer–titanium nanocomposite system produced by DLP. Due to oxygen-induced charge redistribution in titanium nanoparticles and band bending effects, the EWF may be slightly elevated [18, 19]. The higher work function values detected in samples 7 and 8 may therefore reflect a more oxidized or less conductive surface state. Although electron work function is known to influence biological interactions,

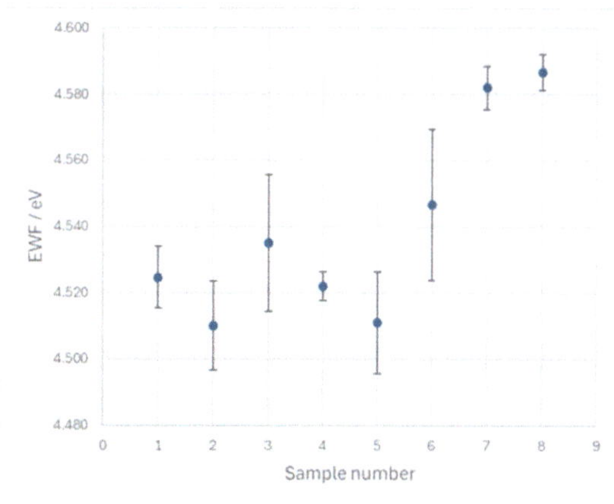

Fig. 8. EWF values of DLP-printed titanium nanocomposite resin samples

this work does not include experimental biological validation. Therefore, direct correlations between the measured EWF values and biological outcomes cannot be established here and will be addressed in future studies.

6 Finite Element Analysis (FEA)

The finite element analysis presented below is focused on simulating the axial compression of a humerus bone affected by an A2-type distal fracture (see Fig. 9). The model has been elaborated assuming that the fracture was surgically treated by internal fixation of a plate implant with five countersunk screws (3 mm diameter). As shown in Fig. 9 b), the axial compression has been applied to the dark blue proximal patch, while the red patch of the distal articular block has been fixed. The analysis has been repeated by increasing the compression load from 0 (zero) to 50 N in steps of 10 N.

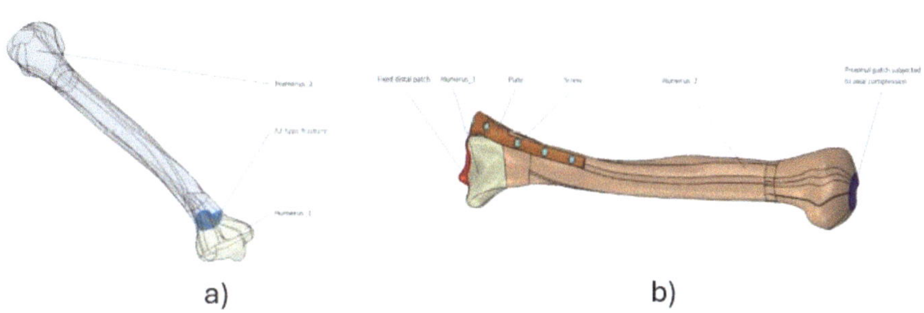

Fig. 9. a) 3D model of the humerus bone affected by an A2-type distal fracture b) Axial compression of the humerus bone affected by an A2-type distal fracture (principle of the FEA)

The finite element model has been prepared with SOLIDWORKS Simulation [20] by adopting the following hypotheses:

- Linear elastic behavior of the model components defined by the physical and mechanical properties listed in Table 1);
- Surface-to-surface contact interactions having the following characteristics (see the denominations presented in Fig. 9 b)):

  - Humerus_1 vs Humerus 2 (fracture region): frictional contact (separation allowed), $\mu = 0.3$;
  - Humerus_1 vs Plate and Humerus_2 vs Plate: frictional contact (separation allowed), $\mu = 0.3$;
  - Humerus_1 vs Screw shaft and Humerus_2 vs Screw shaft: bonded contact;
  - Plate vs Screw head (countersunk): bonded contact;

- Large displacements of the model components to be expected.

Table 1. Physical and mechanical properties of the model components (the upper limits of von Mises equivalent stress represent the yield stress in the case of AISI 316 L or Ti-6Al-4 V, or the ultimate stress in the case of the humerus bone)

Model component	Material	Young's modulus [MPa]	Poisson's ratio [−]	Upper limit of von Mises equivalent stress [MPa]
Humerus_1	Bone	1000	0.300	9
Humerus_2				
Plate	AISI 316 L	193000	0.290	205
Screw	Ti-6Al-4 V	114000	0.342	880

The model has been meshed using 10-node tetrahedral elements. In total, 81657 elements and 127459 nodes have been used in the analysis (Fig. 10).

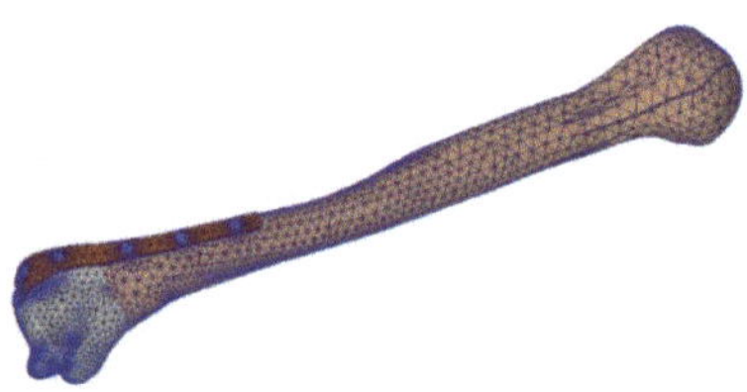

Fig. 10. Finite element mesh used for simulating the axial compression of the humerus bone affected by an A2-type distal fracture

The results of the finite element simulation of the axial compression have shown that the Humerus_2 is the most critical component of the model. As one may notice by analyzing the data listed in Table 2, as well as Fig. 11 a) and b), the maximum value of the von Mises equivalent stress in Humerus_2 exceeds the upper limit defined in Table 1 when the compression force is in the range 30 ÷ 40 N. Because of this lack of stiffness, the movements of the humerus must be restricted in the post-operative stage by a shell made of plaster or fiberglass.

Table 2. Maximum Von Mises Stress in Components Under Axial Compression (results of the finite element analysis)

Compression force [N]	Maximum value of the von Mises equivalent stress in different components of the finite element model [MPa]							
	Humerus_1	Humerus_2	Plate	Screw_1	Screw_2	Screw_3	Screw_4	Screw_5
10	5.0	5.7	112.7	73.6	16.3	51.7	35.6	105.1
20	5.4	6.2	106.3	60.5	21.8	49.7	44.3	96.8
30	6.1	8.2	117.8	57.9	26.4	58.0	56.4	94.2
40	6.9	10.1	115.8	63.1	32.7	59.9	72.3	84.5
50	7.7	12.1	114.9	71.7	39.5	61.7	89.0	76.2

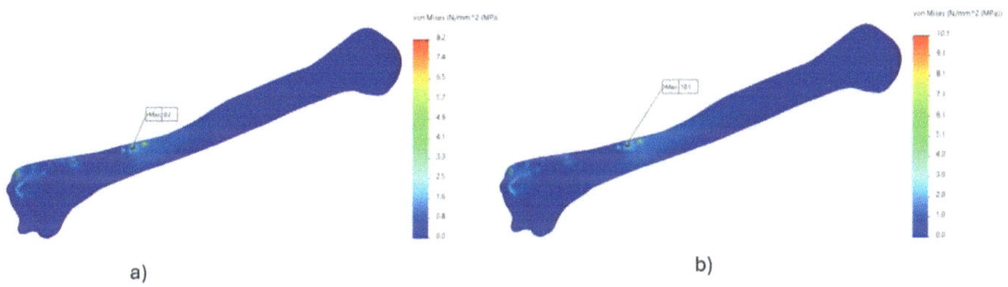

Fig. 11. Distribution of the von Mises equivalent stress in Humerus_1 and Humerus_2 loaded by a compression force of: a) 30 N b) 40 N

7 Conclusions

This study successfully developed and rigorously validated its efficacy as an active interfacial layer for orthopedic fixation systems. A robust material engineering protocol was established, enabling the synthesis and DLP fabrication of a photopolymer matrix reinforced with 10 vol% TiO_2 nanoparticles, while maintaining optimal rheological properties for high-resolution 3D printing. Comprehensive characterization via FTIR and PEES confirmed molecular homogeneity and a highly stable surface energy. The Electron Work Function (EWF) was measured within the narrow range of 4.51–4.59 eV, confirming the material's potential to facilitate optimal bioactive interactions essential for cellular adhesion and osseointegration, however, biological validation is still required to confirm these effects. While the CAD design provided superior geometrical fit (0.1–0.2 mm deviation), the FEA results established the critical biomechanical benchmark, indicating that the structural integrity of the assembly (material + bone) is maintained under axial compression up to 30–40 N. This research, therefore, provides a complete material design methodology that successfully transforms a passive implant into an active system, supported by the dual functionality of the TiO_2 nanocomposite.

Acknowledgment. This work was supported by the ERASMUS + Partnerships for Cooperation and Exchange of Practices (KA220) project titled "Biomedical Innovations through Digital Transformation of Additive Technologies and Knowledge Exchange" — BIOMEDIX (Project No. 2024-1-LV01-KA220-HED-000255929). 0425 project titled "UTCN GLOBE – University without frontiers".

References

1. Donaghy M, Donaghy A, Al-Jaberi H, Ma S (2019) Titanium for orthopedic applications: an overview of surface modification to improve biocompatibility and prevent bacterial biofilm formation. Materials 12(23):3986. https://doi.org/10.3390/ma12233986
2. Christian D, Miguel P, Kley A, Christopher S (2014) TiO_2 anatase with a bandgap in the visible region. Nano Lett 14:6533–6538
3. Al-Dhahir KA, Al-Tameemi N (2024) Review of 3D printing of polyaryletherketone/apatite composites for lattice structures for orthopedic implants. Machines 12(4):1804
4. Manestar D, Maričić S, Komljenović D, Miletić D, Ružić Baršić A, Borović E (2017) Auricular epithesis. Laryngoscope 127(3):574–576
5. Maričić S, Kovačević Pavičić D, Perinić M, Lajnert V (2011) The use of technological documentation in vestibuloplasty fixture plate production. Medicina Fluminensis 47(3):294–298
6. Pato BV et al (2021) Dual-functional nano-functionalized titanium scaffolds to inhibit bacterial growth and enhance osteointegration. Nano 11(10):2634
7. Liu Y, Tang Y, Zhang Y, Ma H (2024) Advances in 3D-printed scaffold technologies for bone defect repair: materials, biomechanics, and clinical prospects. Bioact Mater 35:101740
8. Yanagisawa K, Ovenstone J (1999) Crystallization of anatase from amorphous titania using the hydrothermal technique. J Phy Chem B 103:7781–7787
9. LNCS Homepage. https://www.3ds.com/make/service/3d-printing-service/sla-stereolithography. Last accessed 5 Nov 2025
10. Nam J, Kim M (2024) Advances in materials and technologies for digital light processing 3D printing. Nano Convergence 11(1):45
11. Vitković N et al (2023) Extra-articular distal humerus plate 3D model creation by using the method of anatomical features. Materials 16(15):5409
12. Tavakoli S, Solouk A, Shafiee A (2020) ZnO nanostructures for tissue engineering applications. Nano 10(11):2217
13. Ebrahimi M, Botlagunta A, Ghadiri M, Ghasemi Y, Hasani-Sadrabadi MM (2021) The impact of Zn-doped synthetic polymer materials on bone regeneration: a systematic review. J Appl Biomater Funct Mater 19:123
14. Borș AI (2025) Fourier-transform infrared spectroscopy analysis of 3D-printed dental resins reinforced with yttria-stabilized zirconia nanoparticles. Dentistry journal 13(6):272
15. Vasconcelos D, Costa V, Nunes E, Sabioni A, Gasparon M, Vasconcelos W (2011) Infrared spectroscopy of titania sol-gel coatings on 316L stainless steel. Mater Sci Appl 2:1375–1382
16. Al-Amin M, Dey S, Rashid T, Ashaduzzaman M, Shamsuddin S (2016) Solar assisted photocatalytic degradation of reactive azo dyes in presence of anatase titanium dioxide. Int J Renewable Energy Res 2:14–21

17. Rahim S, Radiman S, Hamzah A (2012) Inactivation of escherichia coli under fluorescent lamp using TiO_2 nanoparticles synthesized via sol gel method. Sains Malaysiana 41:219–224
18. Cieślik K, Wrana D, Rogala M, Rodenbücher C, Szot K, Krok F (2023) The effect of reduction and oxidation processes on the work function of metal oxide crystals: TiO2(110) and SrTiO3(001) case. Crystals 13(7):1052
19. Vella Durai SC, Kumar E, Muthuraj D (2021) Investigations on structural, optical, and impedance spectroscopy studies of titanium dioxide nanoparticles. Bull Chem Soc Ethiop 35:151–160
20. Dassault Systèmes SOLIDWORKS Simulation. https://www.solidworks.com/product/solidworks-simulation. Last accessed 7 Nov 2025

Next-Generation Biocompatibility: Reviewing the Frontier of Novel Materials in Medical AM

Sven Maricic[1,2(✉)] and Mihael Holi[1]

[1] Faculty of Engineering, Juraj Dobrila University of Pula, Negrijeva 6, 52100 Pula, Croatia
smaricic@unipu.hr

[2] Faculty of Medicine, University of Rijeka, Br. Branchetta 20, 51000 Rijeka, Croatia

Abstract. Additive manufacturing in medicine is moving from passive structural replacements toward active, biologically interactive materials that can respond, regenerate, or gradually dissolve after fulfilling their function. This review summarizes studies from 2020–2025 covering four classes of emerging materials: (i) smart and stimuli-responsive systems, including shape-memory polymers and hydrogels that change form or properties in response to heat, acidity, or moisture; (ii) regenerative bioinks and hydrogels, both natural and synthetic, developed to enhance printability, cell survival, and vascular growth; (iii) bioresorbable metals and composites, such as magnesium and zinc alloys, processed by additive manufacturing and modified to maintain strength while controlling the rate of degradation inside the body; and (iv) nano-functionalized feedstocks in which nanoparticles of silver, copper, zinc oxide, graphene, or hydroxyapatite provide antibacterial, electrical, or bone-stimulating functions. The paper discusses the balance between printability and biocompatibility, the stability of new materials during sterilization, and their mechanical durability compared with biological tissues. Regulatory aspects for variable additive manufacturing batches and biologically active materials are also reviewed. The discussion concludes with three guiding questions for clinical adoption: Is it printable? Is it safe? Is it superior to conventional titanium or polyetheretherketone implants? Bioresorbable magnesium systems and smart polymer platforms appear closest to near-term clinical use as process control and material standards advance.

Keywords: 4D printing · bioinks · bioresorbable metals · nanocomposites · antibacterial nanoparticles · process innovation

1 Introduction

The evolution of materials used in medical additive manufacturing can be divided into two main phases: the period of passive materials and the current transition toward active materials. Early medical applications of additive manufacturing focused on passive load-bearing implants such as titanium alloys and polyetheretherketone. These materials were selected for their mechanical stability, corrosion resistance, and biocompatibility, but their role was purely structural. They restored shape and strength without providing any biological stimulus or interaction with the surrounding tissue.

F. Górski et al. (Eds.): MANUFACTURING 2026, LNME, pp. 172–184, 2026.
https://doi.org/10.1007/978-3-032-23089-8_14

Over the past decade, research has moved decisively toward active materials that respond to or influence biological processes. These materials are designed to adapt their mechanical or chemical behavior under physiological conditions, release therapeutic agents, or gradually resorb once healing is complete. Additive manufacturing has enabled precise control of internal architecture, porosity, and composition, allowing researchers to combine geometry-based optimization with biological functionality at the material level.

The clinical motivation for this shift is clear. Conventional permanent implants often fail to integrate fully with host tissue and can cause stress shielding, chronic inflammation, bacterial colonization, and the eventual need for secondary removal surgery. Active materials address these challenges by promoting cell adhesion, vascularization, and controlled degradation, thereby reducing long-term complications and improving patient outcomes.

The objective of this review is to analyze research published between 2020 and 2025 that explores the next generation of biologically interactive materials produced by additive manufacturing. The discussion is organized around four material capability classes: smart and stimuli-responsive systems, regenerative bioinks and hydrogels, bioresorbable metals and composites, and nano-functionalized feedstocks. Emphasis is placed on how each class advances the transition from structural replacement to functional regeneration and how these developments shape the future of medical additive manufacturing.

2 Methodology

The methodological approach aimed to provide a comprehensive and balanced overview of recent developments in biologically interactive materials produced by additive manufacturing. The review focuses on publications that demonstrate experimental validation or early clinical applicability between 2020 and 2025. All records were identified, screened, and categorized by material capability rather than chemical composition to highlight functional behavior relevant to medical use.

The literature search was conducted across three major databases: PubMed, Scopus, and Google Scholar. Each was queried using predefined keyword strings adapted from previous reviews. The primary search terms included "4D printing," "bioinks," "hydrogels," "smart polymers," "bioresorbable additive manufacturing," "biodegradable metal," and "nanocomposite feedstocks." Boolean operators and quotation marks refined the results and eliminated unrelated records. Only articles written in English and published within the defined five-year period were considered.

To ensure relevance, inclusion criteria required that each study involve materials in the experimental stage-demonstrating laboratory-scale synthesis, printing, or biological testing-or in the early clinical phase, where prototypes or implants were evaluated in vitro or in vivo. Exclusion criteria removed theoretical studies without material validation and research unrelated to medical applications. All eligible articles were grouped into four categories: smart and stimuli-responsive systems, regenerative bioinks and hydrogels, bioresorbable metals and composites, and nano-functionalized feedstocks. In total, 49 publications met the inclusion criteria and were selected for analysis.

3 Key Categories of Material Classes for Additive Manufacturing

The growing complexity of clinical needs has driven additive manufacturing toward materials that not only replicate anatomical structure but also participate actively in biological processes. Rather than being defined solely by chemical composition, these materials are better understood through the capabilities they provide-responsiveness, regeneration, controlled resorption, or functional enhancement. Grouping by capability highlights the link between a material's behavior and its clinical purpose, offering a clearer perspective than traditional chemistry-based classifications.

This section presents a capability-oriented review of four key categories identified in the recent literature: smart and stimuli-responsive materials, regenerative bioinks and hydrogels, bioresorbable metals and composites, and nano-functionalized feedstocks. Each category is discussed in terms of its underlying concept, major experimental advances, and relevance to medical applications, emphasizing how additive manufacturing transforms these materials from laboratory prototypes into clinically promising solutions.

3.1 Smart and Stimuli-Responsive Materials (4D Printing)

Additive manufacturing has expanded beyond static design toward materials that can actively transform their shape or physical state after printing. The concept of four-dimensional (4D) printing introduces time as a functional parameter, enabling printed structures to change configuration or mechanical properties when exposed to heat, moisture, light, or pH variations. Such stimuli-responsive behavior allows printed implants or scaffolds to adapt dynamically to physiological conditions rather than remaining fixed once implanted [1, 2].

The foundation of this field lies in shape-memory polymers, which can be temporarily deformed and subsequently recover their original geometry when triggered by temperature or other stimuli. Recent studies describe applications such as self-expanding vascular stents, adaptive sutures, and soft-tissue scaffolds that respond to body temperature [3–5]. Composites combining polymers with reinforcing or conductive fillers have further improved recovery accuracy, durability, and activation control [6, 7]. Hydrogels with reversible swelling and deswelling behavior add a complementary dimension: they can regulate drug release, mimic tissue movement, or provide micro-actuation in minimally invasive devices [8, 9] (Fig. 1).

Emerging 4D-printing strategies couple smart materials with precise digital fabrication methods such as direct-ink-writing, fused-filament fabrication, or digital-light processing. These combinations have produced bioinspired constructs capable of controlled deformation, enhanced cell compatibility, and programmable healing functions [10–12]. The current challenge lies in balancing responsiveness with mechanical reliability: the same flexibility that allows movement can reduce load-bearing strength. Research continues to optimize polymer crosslinking, filler dispersion, and activation thresholds to achieve clinically usable smart devices [13–15].

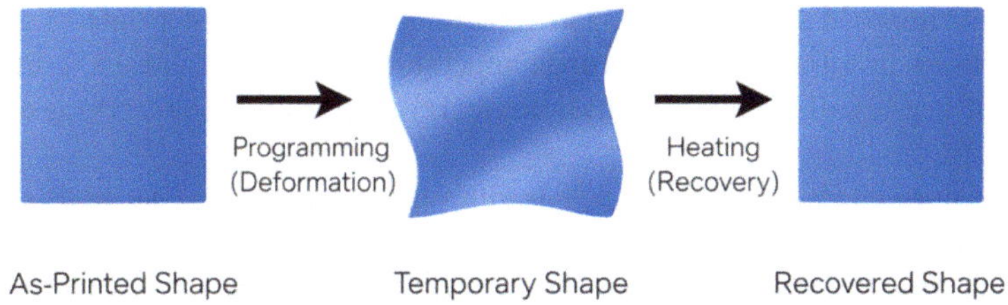

Fig. 1. 4D-printed shape-memory polymer showing programmed and recovered shapes after heating.

3.2 Regenerative Bioinks and Hydrogels

The transition from structural scaffolds to regenerative bioinks marks one of the most transformative advances in bioprinting. These materials are designed not only to provide mechanical support but also to actively promote tissue growth and cellular integration. Hydrogels, composed of hydrophilic polymer networks, are central to this concept because they can encapsulate cells, biomolecules, and nutrients while maintaining a tissue-like microenvironment [16, 17] (Fig. 2).

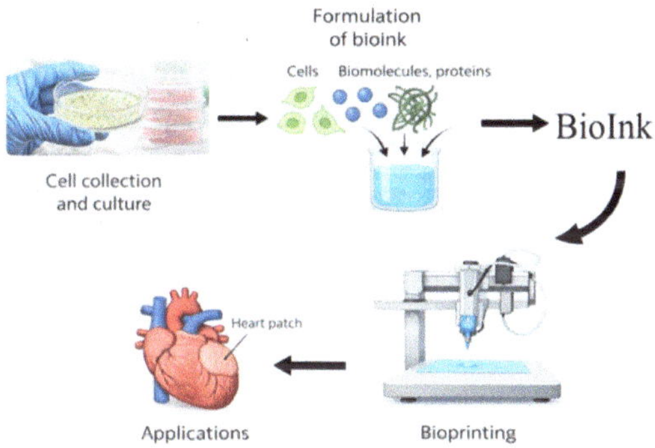

Fig. 2. Workflow of bioprinting using cell-laden bioink from cell collection to tissue application.

Natural polymers such as alginate, collagen, and chitosan remain the most widely studied due to their biocompatibility and similarity to the extracellular matrix. However, their mechanical weakness and variability between sources often limit reproducibility. Synthetic alternatives-including PEG, PVA, and PLGA-based hydrogels-offer superior print fidelity and tunable degradation but may require surface modification to improve cell adhesion [18–20]. Hybrid formulations that combine natural and synthetic components have therefore emerged as an effective compromise, uniting printability with biological performance [21, 22].

A major technical focus lies in the development of cell-laden bioinks, where living cells are incorporated directly into printable matrices. Maintaining cell viability under high extrusion pressures and shear forces remains a central challenge [23, 24]. Optimizing viscosity, nozzle geometry, and crosslinking kinetics has been shown to significantly improve survival rates and functional maturation of printed tissues. For instance, photo-crosslinkable GelMA and temperature-sensitive PLGA-PEG-PLGA systems enable gentle solidification at physiological conditions while preserving embedded cells [25, 26].

Recent research also emphasizes self-healing and stimuli-responsive hydrogels capable of remodeling or releasing bioactive factors in response to local environmental cues [27, 28]. Thermoresponsive nanogels and injectable hydrogels have shown promise for minimally invasive delivery of regenerative materials, combining adaptability with precise control of degradation and diffusion [29, 30]. Collectively, these innovations are redefining the role of bioprinting materials-from passive structural fillers to dynamic bioactive systems that guide regeneration and restore tissue functionality.

3.3 Bioresorbable Metals and Composites

Bioresorbable metals have redefined the purpose of temporary implants by introducing materials that gradually dissolve once healing is complete. This eliminates the need for secondary removal surgeries and reduces long-term complications associated with permanent hardware. Among candidate systems, magnesium (Mg) and zinc (Zn) alloys are the most extensively studied because they combine mechanical strength with natural metabolic compatibility [31, 32].

Additive manufacturing processes, particularly laser powder bed fusion (LPBF), have enabled the precise control of porosity and microstructure necessary to tailor mechanical and corrosion properties. WE43 and ZM10 magnesium alloys produced by LPBF show excellent osseointegration and tunable degradation in both in vitro and in vivo models [33, 34]. However, the key challenge remains the rapid corrosion rate of Mg-based implants in physiological environments. Excess hydrogen evolution and pH shifts can impair tissue regeneration, prompting extensive work on coatings and alloy modifications [35, 36] (Fig. 3).

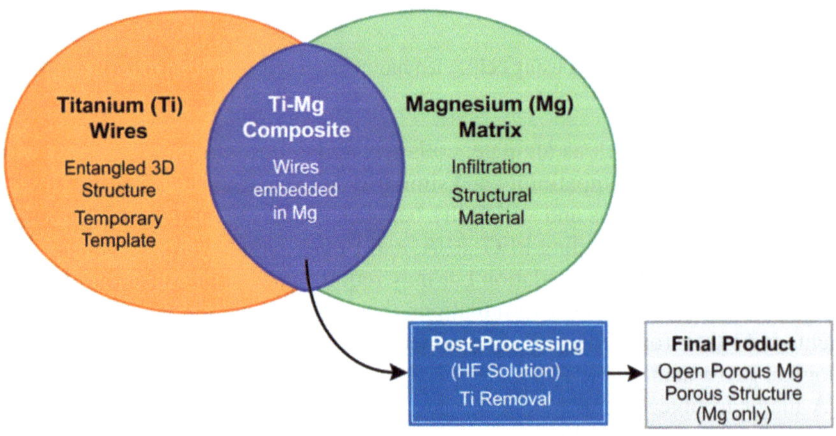

Fig. 3. Stepwise fabrication and structure of a porous magnesium scaffold using a Ti wire template and chemical removal process, resulting in an interconnected bioresorbable framework.

Recent approaches include fluoride, carbonate, and polymeric surface coatings that act as diffusion barriers, slowing degradation while improving biocompatibility [37, 38]. Composite routes, such as Mg-MgF_2 systems or Mg reinforced with rare-earth elements, provide additional strength and corrosion resistance [39, 40]. Environmental studies of calcareous deposition further inform how surface chemistry influences electrochemical stability and cell adhesion [41, 42].

Together, these strategies illustrate a shift from simple mechanical optimization to biologically adaptive control of resorption kinetics. The current frontier lies in balancing structural integrity during healing with predictable degradation afterward-a design equilibrium that continues to drive clinical translation of Mg- and Zn-based additively manufactured implants.

3.4 Nanomaterial-Functionalized Feedstocks

Nanomaterial-functionalized feedstocks represent a new generation of printable materials in which standard polymers are enhanced with nanoparticles to introduce specific physical or biological functionalities. Rather than serving solely as structural matrices, these nanocomposites exploit the high surface area, electrical conductivity, and antibacterial potential of nanofillers to create materials with multifunctional performance [43, 44] (Fig. 4).

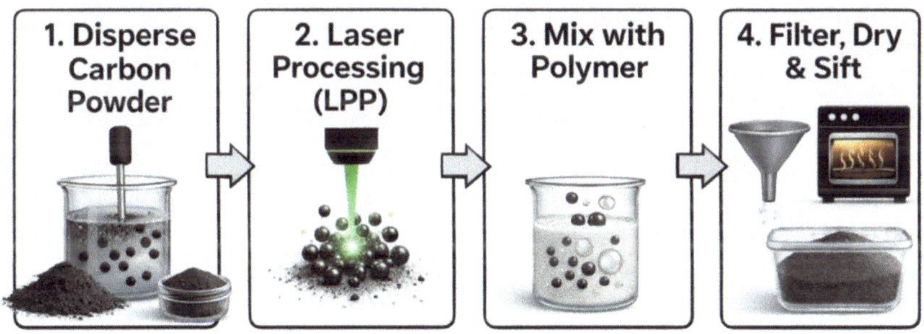

Fig. 4. Process sequence for preparing nanomaterial-functionalized polymer feedstocks.

Antibacterial modification remains one of the most significant drivers of this field. The incorporation of metallic nanoparticles-such as silver, copper, or titanium dioxide-into polymer filaments effectively inhibits bacterial colonization and biofilm formation on medical implants and prosthetics [45, 46]. Optimizing filler dispersion and concentration is critical, as excessive nanoparticle loading can compromise filament integrity and lead to nozzle abrasion during printing. Recent work demonstrates that post-processing and re-extrusion can alter the spatial distribution of nanoparticles, thereby changing the antibacterial response of printed parts [46].

Parallel progress has occurred in electrically conductive nanocomposites, particularly those reinforced with carbon nanotubes or graphene derivatives. These materials combine printability with the electrical and thermal properties required for neural interfaces, biosensors, and tissue-stimulating scaffolds [47, 48, 49]. Controlled orientation of conductive fillers during extrusion has enabled anisotropic networks that support signal transmission while maintaining flexibility. Studies also highlight the potential for hybrid reinforcement-mixing graphene with additional functional nanofillers-to achieve simultaneous mechanical strength and bioactivity [47, 48, 49].

Recent reviews emphasize the need for standardized evaluation of nanocomposite safety and long-term stability, as the leaching of nanoparticles or their accumulation in tissues remains insufficiently characterized [43]. Despite these challenges, nanomaterial-functionalized feedstocks are emerging as versatile building blocks for the next generation of active biomedical devices, bridging the gap between mechanical design, biological performance, and electronic functionality.

4 Critical Analysis: The Gap Between Lab and Clinic

Although additive manufacturing has enabled a remarkable diversity of biointeractive materials, translation into clinical use remains limited. Most studies still demonstrate proof-of-concept at laboratory scale rather than validated, sterilizable, and mechanically reliable implants. The following discussion highlights three recurring barriers that separate experimental success from medical feasibility: printability versus biocompatibility, sterilization stability, and mechanical integrity (Table 1).

Table 1. Typical trade-offs between printability and biocompatibility across emerging AM materials.

Material class	High printability factors	Biocompatibility advantages	Main limitation
Thermoplastic polymers (PCL, PLA) [16, 18]	Stable extrusion, sharp resolution	Good mechanical strength, U.S. Food and Drug Administration (FDA) familiarity	Limited cell adhesion, poor bioactivity
Natural hydrogels (alginate, collagen, chitosan) [16–18, 20]	Mild printing conditions	High cell viability, ECM mimicry	Weak mechanical stability, shape collapse
Synthetic hydrogels (PEG, PLGA, PVA) [19, 24, 25]	Tunable viscosity, crosslinkable	Adjustable degradation rate	Often cytotoxic precursors, poor adhesion
Shape-memory polymers [3–6, 15]	Precise deformation control	Dynamic response to temperature/pH	Difficult sterilization, fatigue degradation
Bioresorbable metals (Mg, Zn) [31–36]	High strength, precision LPBF	Gradual resorption, bone-like modulus	Rapid corrosion, hydrogen release

Printability versus biocompatibility represents the first and most persistent trade-off. Materials optimized for cell adhesion, nutrient diffusion, or degradation control often exhibit rheological properties incompatible with precise layer deposition. Hydrogels rich in biological macromolecules, for instance, provide an excellent microenvironment for living cells but lack the viscosity and crosslinking speed needed for stable three-dimensional printing. Conversely, polymers engineered for sharp dimensional accuracy-such as high-molecular-weight PEG or PCL composites-may require elevated extrusion temperatures or solvents that reduce cell viability. Achieving the correct balance between fluidity, shear stability, and post-printing crosslinking remains a central engineering challenge in biofabrication.

A second limitation concerns sterilization stability. Before any material can enter a clinical environment, it must withstand sterilization through autoclaving, ethylene oxide exposure, or gamma irradiation without losing structural or functional integrity. Many of the new polymeric and hydrogel systems suffer from thermal degradation, chain scission, or loss of responsive behavior after standard sterilization cycles. Similarly, magnesium-based alloys can undergo accelerated corrosion or surface oxidation when exposed to steam or high-energy radiation. Recent studies propose alternative low-temperature methods such as plasma treatment, ultraviolet-ozone exposure, and supercritical CO_2 sterilization, but their scalability and regulatory acceptance are still under evaluation [17, 31, 36]. Establishing standardized sterilization protocols specific to additively manufactured biointeractive materials remains an unmet requirement for clinical translation.

Finally, mechanical integrity must be reconsidered in the context of porous and resorbable architectures. Additive manufacturing enables intricate lattice structures that mimic cancellous bone, yet their fatigue life is often below that of the tissues they aim to replace. The interplay between pore geometry, anisotropy, and degradation introduces complex stress distributions that traditional mechanical models fail to predict accurately. For magnesium and zinc alloys, degradation-driven pitting can act as premature crack initiators, while for polymeric scaffolds, swelling and relaxation cycles reduce load-bearing capacity over time. Integrating in-situ monitoring, computational modeling, and accelerated aging tests into the design process is increasingly seen as essential to ensure predictable long-term behavior [13, 43].

Collectively, these factors underline that material innovation alone does not guarantee clinical readiness. Bridging the laboratory-to-clinic divide will require harmonized approaches that couple biological performance with manufacturability, sterilization robustness, and mechanical reliability-criteria that must evolve in parallel with the materials themselves.

5 Regulatory and Standardization Challenges

Despite rapid progress in biointeractive additive manufacturing, regulatory and standardization frameworks have not yet adapted to the dynamic nature of these materials. Traditional certification methods-developed for homogenous, mass-produced implants-struggle to accommodate the intrinsic variability introduced by digital design, layer-wise fabrication, and biologically active composition. Two main issues define this challenge: the batch inconsistency of printed parts and the uncertain classification of “active” or “living” medical materials within existing approval systems (Table 2).

Table 2. Regulatory and standardization challenges for biointeractive medical additive manufacturing.

Challenge	Why it occurs in AM	What regulators/standards typically require	Practical mitigation
Process variability / part-to-part inconsistency	Layer-wise fabrication and sensitivity to parameter drift causes variation in porosity, microstructure, and surface chemistry	Defined process window, traceability, documented quality management (e.g., ISO 13485)	In-line monitoring, digital quality logs, parameter locking [13, 43]
Lack of standardized test methods for biointeractive materials	Smart/biological functions evolve over time and are not covered by classic static tests	Validated mechanical/biological test protocols including time-dependence	Time-resolved testing, accelerated aging, functional performance endpoints [13, 43]
Sterilization-induced property changes	Polymers/hydrogels and Mg systems can degrade or change behavior after sterilization	Evidence that sterilization preserves safety and performance	Low-temperature sterilization routes; post-sterilization characterization [17, 31, 36]
Nanoparticle safety and leaching uncertainty	Nanofillers can migrate or release ions; long-term exposure data limited	Toxicology, release testing, long-term biocompatibility evidence	Controlled dispersion, barrier coatings, leachate testing [43, 45, 46]
Classification ambiguity (device–drug–biologic overlap)	Cell-laden and bioactive systems may act as combined products	Clear product classification, risk management, clinical evidence	Early regulatory consultation; define intended use and mode of action [13, 43]

The batch problem arises from the fundamental characteristics of additive manufacturing. Each printed component, even when generated from the same digital model, can differ in microstructure, porosity, and surface chemistry due to small variations in laser power, layer thickness, or environmental conditions. Conventional quality-control standards, designed for casting or machining, rely on representative batch testing-an approach unsuitable for layer-by-layer fabrication where every part is effectively unique. In the literature, researchers have proposed in-line monitoring and digital twin frameworks that capture real-time process parameters to establish traceable production records [13, 43]. Such approaches could serve as digital equivalents of batch certificates, but they remain in early stages of validation and require alignment with international standards such as ISO/ASTM 52920 and ISO 13485 for medical device manufacturing. Without these mechanisms, reproducibility and certification continue to represent the most significant regulatory bottlenecks for medical AM.

The second major issue involves the evolving FDA and MDR regulatory landscape. Both the U.S. Food and Drug Administration and the European Medical Device Regulation currently classify materials according to traditional categories: inert polymers, resorbable metals, or biologically derived tissues. However, emerging additively manufactured systems-such as cell-laden hydrogels, stimuli-responsive polymers, and degradable magnesium alloys-do not fit cleanly into these definitions. For instance, a scaffold that gradually degrades while releasing bioactive molecules or hosting living cells can simultaneously function as a device, drug, and biologic. This hybrid nature complicates risk assessment, labeling, and clinical trial requirements. Recent guidance from the FDA's Center for Devices and Radiological Health emphasizes the need for device-specific additive manufacturing process validation, while the MDR framework introduces post-market surveillance obligations for custom and patient-specific implants. Nevertheless, no unified protocol yet exists for certifying "active" or "living" materials whose performance may evolve after implantation.

The regulatory path forward will depend on a closer integration between material scientists, bioengineers, and policy makers. Establishing reproducibility metrics, digital quality logs, and adaptive testing procedures will be essential for bridging the gap between innovation and compliance. As additive manufacturing continues to blur the boundary between materials and biology, future standards must evolve to evaluate not only how a device is made, but how it behaves, adapts, and interacts with the human body over time.

6 Future Perspectives

Near-term clinical adoption appears most plausible for bioresorbable Mg/Zn platforms and selected smart polymer systems, where core processing routes and performance endpoints are becoming more standardized [31–38]. Progress will depend on integrating in-line monitoring, digital quality records, and validated time-dependent testing to reduce variability between builds and to support certification of biointeractive functions [13, 43]. For regenerative hydrogels and nano-functionalized feedstocks, broader translation will likely require stronger long-term safety evidence (e.g., nanoparticle leaching and degradation products) and sterilization-robust formulations suitable for scalable manufacturing workflows [17, 43, 46]. Ultimately, the field's success will be determined by whether emerging materials can consistently satisfy three adoption criteria: printability, safety, and clear clinical advantage over established titanium or polyetheretherketone solutions.

7 Conclusion

Medical additive manufacturing is shifting from passive structural implants toward biointeractive materials designed to respond, regenerate, or resorb after healing. Across the reviewed literature (2020–2025), four capability-driven categories dominate: (i) smart and stimuli-responsive systems, (ii) regenerative bioinks and hydrogels, (iii) bioresorbable metals and composites, and (iv) nano-functionalized feedstocks. Despite strong laboratory progress, clinical translation remains constrained by reproducibility, sterilization stability, and long-term mechanical integrity in porous and time-evolving architectures.

Most 4D polymer systems still require careful tuning of actuation versus mechanical reliability and fatigue resistance to meet implant-level demands. Bioink performance is largely governed by rheology and crosslinking kinetics, which directly trade off print fidelity against cell survival during extrusion. For Mg/Zn systems, corrosion control is the primary limiter; coatings and alloying remain the dominant levers to stabilize degradation and reduce hydrogen evolution. For nanocomposites, filler dispersion and manufacturability limits (e.g., filament integrity and nozzle wear) frequently constrain antibacterial performance and repeatability. Regulatory readiness increasingly depends on process traceability and standardized evidence packages rather than material novelty alone.

Acknowledgments. This work was supported by the Erasmus + 2024-1-LV01-KA220-HED-000255929 project BioMedix. The authors gratefully acknowledge the support of the BioMedix consortium and partner institutions for providing the collaborative framework and technical resources that contributed to this research.

References

1. Chu H et al (2020) 4D printing: a review on recent progresses. Micromachines 11(9):796. https://doi.org/10.3390/mi11090796
2. Kantaros A (2023) 4D printing: technology overview and smart materials utilized. J Mechatronics Robot 7(1):1–14. https://doi.org/10.3844/jmrsp.2023.1.14
3. Dayyoub T, Maksimkin AV, Filippova OV, Tcherdyntsev VV, Telyshev DV (2022) Shape memory polymers as smart materials: a review. Polymers 14(17):3511. https://doi.org/10.3390/polym14173511
4. Zhao W, Yue C, Liu L, Liu Y, Leng J (2022) Research progress of shape memory polymer and 4D printing in biomedical application. Adv Healthc Mater:2201975. https://doi.org/10.1002/adhm.202201975
5. Pisani S, Genta I, Modena T, Dorati R, Benazzo M, Conti B (2022) Shape-memory polymers hallmarks and their biomedical applications in the form of nanofibers. Int J Mol Sci 23(3):1290. https://doi.org/10.3390/ijms23031290
6. Khalid MY, Arif ZU, Noroozi R, Zolfagharian A, Bodaghi M (2022) 4D printing of shape memory polymer composites: a review on fabrication techniques, applications and future perspectives. J Manuf Process 81:759–797. https://doi.org/10.1016/j.jmapro.2022.07.035
7. Zeng C, Liu L, Hu Y, Bian W, Leng J, Liu Y (2022) A viscoelastic constitutive model for shape memory polymer composites: micromechanical modeling, numerical implementation and application in 4D printing. Mech Mater 169:104301. https://doi.org/10.1016/j.mechmat.2022.104301
8. Champeau M, Heinze DA, Viana TN, de Souza ER, Chinellato AC, Titotto S (2020) 4D printing of hydrogels: a review. Adv Funct Mater 30(31):1910606. https://doi.org/10.1002/adfm.201910606
9. Malekmohammadi S et al (2021) Smart and biomimetic 3D and 4D printed composite hydrogels. Biomedicine 9(11):1537. https://doi.org/10.3390/biomedicines9111537
10. Wang Y, Cui H, Esworthy T, Mei D, Wang Y, Zhang LG (2022) Emerging 4D printing strategies for next-generation tissue regeneration and medical devices. Adv Mater 34(20):2109198. https://doi.org/10.1002/adma.202109198

11. Razzaq MY, Gonzalez-Gutierrez J, Mertz G, Ruch D, Schmidt DF, Westermann S (2022) 4D printing of multicomponent shape-memory polymer formulations. Appl Sci 12(15):7880. https://doi.org/10.3390/app12157880
12. Du C, Liu J, Fikhman DA, Dong KS, Monroe MBB (2022) Shape memory polymer foams with phenolic acid-based antioxidant and antimicrobial properties. Front Bioeng Biotechnol 10:961358. https://doi.org/10.3389/fbioe.2022.809361
13. Mahmood A, Akram T, Chen H, Chen S (2022) On the evolution of additive manufacturing (3D/4D printing) technologies. Polymers 14(21):4698. https://doi.org/10.3390/polym14214698
14. Hu L, Gao Y, Serpe MJ (2022) Smart stimuli-responsive polymers, films and gels. Wiley. https://doi.org/10.1002/9783527832385.ch2
15. Zhang J, Yin Z, Ren L, Liu Q, Yang X, Zhou X (2022) Advances in 4D printed shape memory polymers. Adv Mater Technol 7(9):2101568. https://doi.org/10.1002/admt.202101568
16. Ramiah P, du Toit LC, Choonara YE, Kondiah PPD, Pillay V (2020) Hydrogel-based bioinks for 3D bioprinting. Front Mater 7:76. https://doi.org/10.3389/fmats.2020.00076
17. Gómez-Florit M et al (2020) Natural-based hydrogels for tissue engineering. Molecules 25(23):5858. https://doi.org/10.3390/molecules25245858
18. Smandri A, Nordin A, Hwei NM, Chin KY, Abd Aziz I, Fauzi MB (2020) Natural 3D-printed bioinks. Polymers 12(8):1782. https://doi.org/10.3390/polym12081782
19. Zhang K, Xue K, Loh XJ (2021) Thermo-responsive hydrogels. Gels 7(2):77. https://doi.org/10.3390/gels7030077
20. Rijal G (2023) Bioinks of natural biomaterials. Bioengineering 10(6):705. https://doi.org/10.3390/bioengineering10060705
21. Ouyang L et al (2020) Complementary network bioinks. Science Advances 6(37):eabc5529. https://doi.org/10.1126/sciadv.abc5529. Rahman M, Dutta NK, Choudhury NR (2020) Magnesium alloys with tunable interfaces. Front Bioeng Biotechnol 8:564. https://doi.org/10.3389/fbioe.2020.00564
22. Kim H, Jang J, Cho D-W (2022) Multicomponent bioinks for printing liver tissues. Front Bioeng Biotechnol 10:764682. https://doi.org/10.3389/fbioe.2022.764682
23. Yin Y, Hu B, Yuan X, Cai L, Gao H, Yang Q (2020) Nanogels for biomedical applications. Pharmaceutics 12(3):290. https://doi.org/10.3390/pharmaceutics12030290
24. López-Cano JJ et al (2021) Thermo-responsive PLGA-PEG-PLGA hydrogels. Pharmaceutics 13(2):234. https://doi.org/10.3390/pharmaceutics13020234
25. Chatterjee S, Hui PC-L (2021) Stimuli-responsive hydrogels. Polymers 13(13):2086. https://doi.org/10.3390/polym13132086
26. Fan L et al (2020) Self-healing hydrogels. Front Bioeng Biotechnol 8:654. https://doi.org/10.3389/fbioe.2020.00654
27. Devi VKA, Shyam R, Palaniappan A, Jaiswal AK, Oh T-II, Nathanael AJ (2021) Self-healing hydrogels. Polymers 13(21):3782. https://doi.org/10.3390/polym13213782
28. Ghaeini-Hesaroeiye S, Razmi Bagtash H, Boddohi S, Vasheghani-Farahani E, Jabbari E (2020) Thermoresponsive nanogels. Gels 6(3):20. https://doi.org/10.3390/gels6030020
29. Wang M, Li W, Hao J et al (2022) Molecularly cleavable bioinks. Nat. Commun. 13:3317. https://doi.org/10.1038/s41467-022-31002-2
30. Zhou H, Liang B, Jiang H, Deng Z, Yu K (2021) Magnesium-based biomaterials. J Magnesium Alloys 9:779–804. https://doi.org/10.1016/j.jma.2021.03.004
31. Liu J, Liu B, Min S et al (2022) WE43 scaffolds by LPBF. Bioact Mater 16:301–319. https://doi.org/10.1016/j.bioactmat.2022.02.020
32. Sasaki M, Xu W, Koga Y et al (2022) Parylene-coated Mg stents. Materials 15:3132. https://doi.org/10.3390/ma15093132
33. Dvorsky D, Kubasek J, Jablonska E, Vojtech D (2020) Mg-MgF_2 composites. J Alloys Compd 825:154016. https://doi.org/10.1016/j.jallcom.2020.154016

34. Liu D, Yang D, Li X, Hu S (2019) Mechanical properties, corrosion resistance and biocompatibilities of degradable Mg–RE alloys: a review. J Mater Res Technol 8:1538–1549. https://doi.org/10.1016/j.jmrt.2018.08.003
35. Popa M, Stefan LM, Prelipcean AM, Drob SI, Anastasescu M (2022) Carbonate coatings for Mg. Corros Sci 209:110775. https://doi.org/10.1016/j.corsci.2022.110775
36. Peng W, Chen Y, Fan H, Chen S, Wang H, Song X (2023) PLLA/MgF_2 coatings. Materials 16:682. https://doi.org/10.3390/ma16020682
37. Antoniać I, Miculescu M, Manescu V et al (2022) Magnesium alloys in orthopedics Materials. Materials (Basel) 15:1148. https://doi.org/10.3390/ma15031148
38. Weng W, Biesiekierski A, Li Y, Dargusch M, Wen C (2021) Rare earth elements in Mg alloys. Acta Biomater 130:80–97. https://doi.org/10.1016/j.actbio.2021.06.004
39. Carre C, Zanibellato A, Jeannin M, Sabot R, Gunkel-Grillon P (2020) Calcareous deposition. Environ Chem Lett 18:1193–1208. https://doi.org/10.1007/s10311-020-01002-z
40. Cai S, Wu C, Yang W, Liang W, Yu H, Liu L (2020) Surface modification for cell adhesion. Nanotechnol Rev 9:971–989. https://doi.org/10.1515/ntrev-2020-0076
41. Rahman M, Islam KS, Dip TM et al (2024) Nanomaterial-based additive manufacturing. Prog Addit Manuf 9:1197–1224. https://doi.org/10.1007/s40964-023-00514-8
42. Alli YA et al (2023) Influence of nanocomposites in extrusion-based 3D printing: a review. Hybrid Adv 3:100069. https://doi.org/10.1016/j.hybadv.2023.100069
43. Silva M, Pinho IS, Covas JA et al (2021) Graphene polymer nanocomposites. Funct Compos Mater 2:8. https://doi.org/10.1186/s42252-021-00020-6
44. Pinho AC et al (2025) Antibacterial nanocomposite filaments. Polymers 17(2):171. https://doi.org/10.3390/polym17020171
45. Hisham M et al (2024) Additive manufacturing of carbon nanocomposites for structural applications. J Mater Res Technol 28:4674–4693. https://doi.org/10.1016/j.jmrt.2024.01.049
46. Wu Y, An C, Guo Y (2023) 3D printed graphene composites. Materials 16(16):5681. https://doi.org/10.3390/ma16165681
47. Iqbal AA et al (2024) Graphene (GNP) reinforced 3D printing nanocomposites: an advanced structural perspective. Heliyon 10(7):e28771. https://doi.org/10.1016/j.heliyon.2024.e28771
48. Ashtiani HRR (2025) Mechanical and antibacterial performance of TiO_2 nanoparticle reinforced polymer nanocomposites fabricated via additive manufacturing. J Reinf Plast Compos. https://doi.org/10.1177/00219983251393494

Author Index

F. Górski et al. (Eds.): MANUFACTURING 2026, LNME, pp. 185–186, 2026.
https://doi.org/10.1007/978-3-032-23089-8

MIX
Papier aus verantwortungsvollen Quellen
Paper from responsible sources
FSC® C105338

If you have any concerns about our products,
you can contact us on
ProductSafety@springernature.com

In case Publisher is established outside the EU,
the EU authorized representative is:
Springer Nature Customer Service Center GmbH
Europaplatz 3, 69115 Heidelberg, Germany

Printed by Libri Plureos GmbH
in Hamburg, Germany